When a Lion Speaks
Volume One
The Tears of a Black Man

Curator: Sista Jay Jay

When A Lion Speaks

Copyright © 2024 JoeDrell Sista Jay Jay Benjamin
Editor: Horace Marcell
R.A.G Girl Publishing
All rights reserved.
ISBN: **9798325442803**

When A Lion Speaks

To: My friend Carla
It has been a long journey! Thanks for being a good friend all of these years!! God is still working on us & I am excited about what is yet to come.
Love,
Horace W. Marcell

DEDICATION

This book is dedicated to every black man that has lived, died, and yet to be born.

When A Lion Speaks

CONTENTS

Acknowledgments   i

Introduction   ii

1   Horace Marcell   Pg #1
2   Jerome 'JWritezz' Bradley   Pg #54
3   Foree Shalom   Pg #76
4   Troyeusta TC Apkins   Pg #122
5   Sista Jay Jay   Pg #161

When A Lion Speaks

ACKNOWLEDGMENTS

I would like to acknowledge my stepdad, Kenneth Earl Hines (Brother Kenny) and my grandfather Willie Lankford Stith (Grandpa Najee) and my current stepfather, Jan LaBoo (Pops).
These men have shown me the meaning of love, fatherhood and what a real black man looks like. I thank you for being who you are. It's not about how perfect you are, or were, it's about having a heart of *perfected* love.
Each of you have shown me that through the tears of a black man, he continues to strive for greatness, love, success, integrity, and it is his perseverance, hard and smart work, growth, humbleness, forgiveness, wisdom, that has enabled him to be as powerful as he is, and what the world has yet to see.
Thank you.

INTRODUCTION

I have heard people say on many occasions that black men don't read and to a degree, I agree. However, I realized that it's not that black men don't read, it's that they do not have a desire to read the books that are given to them to read. Let's think about it for a moment, who wants to read how, people are better than them or how they were always the underdog, and there is no triumph in the end, or how they are always wrong, or how they don't have feelings? Okay, let's talk about the books they gave us to read in school, like Mark Twain, although I like his books, my brothers found them boring. I later realized that my brothers were interested in books that spoke to their inner male blackness. You may ask, what is that? Only a black man can really explain it to you but at the same time maybe they won't because that is the one thing that no other race male or female can understand. It is their own language and only they understand it. So, I don't even try to evade their space, however, I do have empathy for the tears that they have not been given permission to release and the pain they have not been given permission to feel and heal from.

So, this book is just that. It is about black men talking to black men, giving each other hope, understanding, empathy, strength, peace, and yes love and permission and although, others may read it, the language within the pages we may not understand, but black men who read it will.

For years now black women have been given permission to embrace their darkest and painful moments in order to heal, and we are soaring to higher heights but how can we healed, soaring women expect to have a productive and successful relationship with our black men, if our black men are not afforded that same opportunity to embrace their trauma and heal from it?

My hope is that after our black men read this book, they will make a decision to embrace their trauma and begin the healing, forgiveness, that is needed to enhance their inner strength, and to know that it is okay to not be okay and not to know it all and to be afraid at times, and not have the answers but what is not okay, is to not do something about it.

Enjoy.

KILLER WORDS

AUTHOR: ELDER HORACE MARCELL

CHAPTER ONE

It was 1:15am, January 29, 2024, when I began to cry out. What happened to my trust? What happened to my faith? My journey has been one full of tears, hurt and fear. But amid the most difficult times, I learned to trust, believe in, and follow the voice of the Almighty God, my Creator. And now here I am through all the trials and tribulation, finding myself despondent and dismayed and at an all-time spiritual low. A lifetime of trials, tribulations, hurt, pain, grief, and tears had finally caught up with me and wore me down. Hear me, I am a Lion! See my tears. I am a Black Man and I do cry.

From the time I was a little boy my life has been plagued with one heartache after another. My fate has been suffering from the lack of family and friends. It has been the pain and reality of one-sided relationships. And when I say relationships, I am not referring to superficial romantic escapades. I am talking about normal everyday relationships that come from having family, friends, teachers, co-workers, social alliances, etc. I am talking about the relationships that every human should be able to experience and enjoy because they are built on the mutuality of love, care, and commitment. But unlike normality, those relationships broke me, ripped me to shreds, and left me hanging on for dear life. But guess what? I'm still standing. Hear me, I am a Lion! See my tears. I am a Black Man and I do cry.

Even in finding my way to the House of God, I have continually been met with jealousy, deceit, hurt, pain, and abuse. That's right, the church, the house of worship. The one place that should be a place of refuge and deliverance and care and concern didn't have a flowing fountain for me to sip from. The one place that should be overflowing with love and compassion didn't have a gusher for me to draw from. What it offered me was cuts and stabs that created a flow of tears that left me damaged and broken. Now I am not saying it has been all bad. I have had some amazing times in the sanctuary among the laity. But behind closed doors, among the leadership, in the trenches that make a church flow, I have certainly had my share of the bad. Hear me, I am a Lion! See my tears. I am a Black Man and I do cry.

Most people around me have no idea the inner sufferings I bear. They cannot see nor feel the hidden sadness, the pain and anguish, the scars, the emotional and psychological struggle. They don't even see the baggage, the weight, the fight, the war within resulting from the war without. When someone suffers physical abuse, they must find ways to hide the scars that are in visible places. They cover the scars that are in places that are normally clothed by shirts, pants, jackets and the like. And of course, they put on the public smile and personification of happiness, comfort, love and joy. Every day until the marks fade away over the course of time, they are reminded daily of their sufferings. The greater tragedy is that some scars never fade completely away. They get lighter and lighter, often to the point of being almost invisible but still present. But in the course of time, the abused learns to live with and to "overlook" the scars. And the scars become constant reminders of the damaged past. But there is also the other side of the coin so to speak. The overcomer, the triumphant, the survivor, the new being that arises out of the ashes of the abused, the defeated, the dead. Hear me, I am a Lion! See my tears. I am a Black Man and I do cry.

What we are about to embark upon is a small peak into several stops along the journey of my life. As we journey, there are a few things that I believe most of us have in common. Our paths are full of ups and downs, good and bad, trials and tribulations, and challenges. What ultimately matters are how we handle each situation and how it affects us in the long run. I will only share a couple of incidents because I want to show and express the power of the tongue. The word of God speaks about the tongue being as sharp as a two-edged sword, cutting both coming and going as I envision it. I want you to journey with me on how two seemingly very small events changed the entire course of my life. Destiny, maybe so. But destiny or not, word hurt is real, and the tongue is the most powerful tool you carry. Well, what about prayer? I'm glad you asked. Prayer is words. So, as you journey with me, please remember that this story is not about the continual series of events and challenges, but the reality of how one event or chain of words can affect life for years to come.

What we do with what we experience is a critical factor in how we live with and handle our present and future situations. Transparency in sharing our dark sides can be overwhelming and yet necessary. It can be overwhelming to take the risk of opening yourself to the world in print, exposing your vulnerability and subjecting yourself to ridicule and judgment. Victims and perpetrators alike are open to the opinions of others based on partial and subjective information supplied through one perspective, one set of eyes. But it is necessary that stories be told because others can learn and grow from the stories and experiences of others. It is necessary because our stories can help others avoid the pits that we have crawled out of. And it is necessary because sometimes sharing brings us deliverance and helps to remove the lingering residue of our bad situations.

I am a teacher by gifting. So, as I share my story you will feel, hear, and learn. As I open these chapters of my life it is my desire that you not only experience the roller coaster but also grasp the lessons along the way that help to develop character and resilience. The Word of God teaches us that God has equipped us with everything that we need to survive this journey called life. It teaches us that we only need faith the size of a mustard seed to make it through every unseen and hidden area, every challenge, every mountain, and every valley in our lives. And finally, it clearly tells us that we have been given "the measure" of faith that we need. In other words, we are always talking about needing more when what we have is already sufficient as given by God. We simply need to grow in the measure that God has given us. Again, it is what we do with what we experience. And so, my story begins. I am a Lion. I do cry. And now…I speak.

There I was about 7 or 8 years old in about the 2nd or 3rd grade when the unthinkable happened. Buckle your seatbelt and let's take a ride. I was born to Josephine Marcell with John Davis by her side. I was the result of an affair between Horace Wilson Hamilton and Josephine Marcell. My Dad, John, was in the Airforce and was involved with my mother at the time of my birth. My biological father was already an absentee father but hopefully not a deadbeat of sorts. Let's fast forward to the unthinkable event, the first life changing moment that I suffered. This moment defined my life in so many ways. In so many ways this moment defied who I am today, both the good and the bad. It created some good character traits and some bad. So, I do not claim to be an angel, but I do work diligently at being the best person that I can possibly be. And so, this moment would prove to be the precursor to the real tragedy of my life. It would become part one of a two event life changer.

It was early that morning and my dad had gone to take my mother to work. Rodney was in his room. Tommy and I were in the kitchen. To this day I don't remember where Mary was. Mary is my mother's oldest child from another man followed by her brother Rodney. They shared the same mother and father. My younger brother, Tommy, was the biological son of my dad. Tommy and I were a dynamic duo. We were up early and hungry. The only one available to fix us something to eat was Rodney. I don't remember the specifics but for whatever reason, that wasn't happening. I decided to do what any good big brother would do. I would fix our breakfast.

I had watched my mother cook eggs so I knew what to do. All I needed was the eggs, a bowl, a skillet, some grease, a fork, and a chair to reach the stove. It was time for the adventure to begin. I was ready to cook my first breakfast. I pulled the chair up to the stove, poured the grease and turned on the fire. I then pulled the chair over to the counter next to the stove to prepare the eggs. I don't know how much time had gone by since turning on the stove, but the oil was good and hot. Yes, it was piping hot. I began the process of cracking the eggs and stirring them in the bowl. Then, from the corner of my eyes as I turned around slightly, I saw him coming down the hallway. It was Rodney, my mother's 2nd born. I turned back and continued stirring the eggs. A moment or so later the unthinkable became my reality.

The voice came. I heard him yelling. It was loud and frightening. As I turned in fear, I saw the hand. One hand reached for the knob and turned the stove up to the max. I could see the flames get bigger right before my eyes, but I had no idea what was happening. With the force of anger, I could hear the screaming. "What do you think you're doing!" No time to think, no time to feel, I just heard those angry words. I heard those words of punishment, those words of judgment. They were the echoing sound of teaching me a lesson. It was a sense of revenge. But what for? What had I done? What was I guilty of? Why was this rage so fierce against me? It was like a voice from the pits of hell. I was just a child. I could not process the tone, the hate, the intention. It simply pierced my soul.

Then I saw the two of them come together on the handle of the pan. The two hands. In a split second it was all over me, the boiling hot grease. The hands released the hot grease into my face, onto my arm, shoulder, and chest. Then there was more screaming. But this time it was the voice coming out of me. The agony, the pain, the bellowing of the hot grease on my skin was crying out for help. But help I did not receive. Instead, I got more angry words. To this day I can't even remember what those words were. I just remember them reinforcing the punishment that had just been thrust upon me. But this time they were joined with the eyes and the face. I could see the anger. I could see the hate. I could feel the effort to diminish me and make my pain and hurt extend beyond the physical damage. Together the voice, the eyes, and the face sang in unison to destroy and belittle me, to make me feel pain beyond measure. Together they formed a satanic vision as they stood over me. They looked down on me and I realized I was helpless. I don't know what other abuse I suffered in that moment as the tears flowed, as the skin burned, and as the fear set in. I just know that they hovered over me in torment as I sank in distress. I can only imagine what was going through Tommy's mind as his eyes witnessed the unthinkable. I can only imagine the shaking of his soul as his ears heard the torture and the torment, the screaming, the yelling, and the crying. He was four years younger than me, and we were one. And although that only made him around four years old, I'm sure that it had some kind of shocking impact on his life. At that tender age we may or may not be able to process but we have lasting visuals that we tend to reflect upon for years to come.

I don't remember what happened next. I only remember my dad arriving and rushing me to the hospital. I don't know how long it was before he arrived at the house. I don't remember the ride to the hospital. Whether I was conscious or unconscious, aware or unaware escapes my memory. I just know that he took me. I do remember arriving at the hospital and being rushed into the emergency room.

From there I was rushed into a private room and packed in ice for several hours. I have no idea what he told the medical staff. I have no idea if they thought to contact child protective services. I don't even remember if I was still crying or if I still felt the pain. But I remember feeling the ice, the cold, the new suffering. Did my injuries and assault even matter to all of the adults who witnessed my state or was I just seen as a medical emergency and released? What I do know is that nothing was done about it. No adult did anything to make sure that I was protected and safe going forward. No one at the hospital asked me what happened. So here I am in the continuum of the unthinkable, finding myself left at the mercy of others once again. What did these voices say about my situation? What conversations took place? Did my dad cover up the truth? What did he tell them? To this day these questions remain unanswered. And since nothing was done about this incident, the abuse would continue for years to come. The adults did not protect me then and they did not protect me from the punishments to come. Welcome to the beginning of my scars.

I believe this was the beginning of my "blocking out." Maybe I was unconscious during much of this event because there are so many gaps. But unconscious or not, I learned to block out most of my childhood after this point. There is so much that I just don't remember because I had trained myself not to. Going forward I would block out most of my childhood because of the tragedy, the hurt, and the pain. It would become the only way that I could survive. It would become the only way that I could deal with myself…block it out.

Next my dad and I would begin the long drive home. Just me and him, my dad. He was the only one I trusted and although I believe he wanted to protect me, he was not the one in charge. I know he felt my pain and I know that there was a lot of confusion in his mind. I could feel the agony as we began to drive. I could sense the confusion in his mind. At that time all of this was subconscious to me, but I would learn later in life that I had spiritual gifting that allowed me to feel and sense what others were dealing with. It was later in life as I grew in my gifting that I was able to consciously analyze the pictures and feelings that still existed within me. As if they had been frozen in time, I was able to revisit the unthinkable and the surrounding emotions and events as I grew spiritually. As more time passed, I would come to understand that my story was designed to be a help to others suffering or having suffered similar fates. The bible tells us that God will never give us more than we can bear. But the question as to why we bear often lingers on in our minds and thoughts for years.

The first stop was to pick my mother up from work. The conversation began as soon as she got into the car and saw me. "What happened to him?" The words were cold and distant as if I were just a thing, as if I didn't really matter. There was no care, no compassion, and no concern for my well-being. It was simply a tone of request for the knowledge of why I was bandaged up. No words came to inquire about my pain, how I felt, or if I needed anything to help my burns. Love and sympathy were completely absent from the tone. The words were hollow and empty.

Discussion followed. And as my mother's voice spoke it was like an extension of Rodney. There I was, the problem. I could feel the anger towards me for making this happen. This was my fault and I got what I deserved. It was as if his voice and eyes and face were looking down on me again, punishing me all over again. While not raised in tone, the anger was very present. I was the disgusting thing, the hated one. I had created a problem and ruined the day. My dad decided to curtail the conversation by telling me that I could have whatever I wanted for dinner. Pizza, I stated as the conversation continued.

Not guilty. That was the verdict for Rodney. It was an accident, and that was the conclusion before the trial. Soon after grabbing the pizza and soda, we arrived back at the house. There the trial began. Rodney takes the stand and Josephine, the judge, asks the question. "What happened?" Rodney proceeds to present his case. "It was an accident. I went into the kitchen; he was standing on a chair, and he had the stove up too high under the hot grease. I turned the stove off, yanked the skillet off the stove and the grease accidentally spilled on him." The verdict came immediately. Innocent. This was just an accident. I had no say, no rebuttal, no expression of what I had suffered. And with this discussion there was never a word or question from Rodney or Josephine as to my pain, how I felt or was I okay. No apology came. I never heard the words, "I'm sorry" from him nor "I'm sorry this happened to you…son" from my mother. They stood their ground as a united force. My dad had no say so. The pizza was all that he could offer to appease the situation and show me some kind of care, support, and love. I knew if he spoke up any more than he did, he would suffer the consequences later that night. He would receive the royal tongue lashing followed by anger and resentment for days to come. He could not stand by my side. He could not be my avenger.

The unspeakable ended with the voices, the eyes and the faces demeaning me once again in unison. They looked down on me and they stared at me with disgust as the conversation in the courtroom (the living room) ended. The hate and the desire for punishment was so clear. It was almost to the point that what was done to me wasn't enough. I deserved more. The pizza didn't bring joy and it didn't bring peace. It only bought an evening with no stove turned on. I have no recollection of where Mary and Tommy were during this part of the tragedy. In my memory their voices were not heard, nor their faces seen. They were simply absent, invisible so to speak. And I was alone, left only to view the distant stare of sympathy from my dad who was powerless. The incident was never spoken of or mentioned in the house again.

Same house, around the same age, part two would take place. Oh…how I hate that residence. The house of horror and the home of no return. It was "family time", or so I thought. Tommy was the only one that loved me unconditionally. My dad loved and cared about me, but he was in bondage. He was trapped by the controls of my mother and confined by the desire and drive to treat everyone the same, to "be fair." He had to find a way to "fit in". Being husband and daddy was his inroad and the object of his life's desire. And time would show that that inroad came at my expense. It benefited the three and hurt the one. And although Tommy and I were as close as Batman and Robin, I was still the outsider as time would soon tell. Yes, Tommy and I were inseparable, a dynamic dual. When you saw one, you saw the other. Our bond was so strong that our names were always called or referred to as one, Alvon, and Tommy. That's right, Alvon. This was the nickname given to me by my dad. I was Alvon Davis, another story for another book.

Back to the conclusion of the matter. We journey to the second life changing moment of my life. As I stated, it was family time…or so I thought. Dad was in the living room and the rest of us were in the kitchen. But for some reason, I really don't remember where Mary was although I believe she was present in the kitchen as well. Tommy and I were playing. I remember being so happy and excited to be spending time with my baby brother as I always did. No matter how much time we spent together, it was never enough, and it was always full of joy. Then the unthinkable happened.

The voice rose up again as if out of nowhere. It came as a sword. It came to cut; it came to hurt. It came as a sarcastic plunder billowing down to smother me with pain. The cynical laughter accompanied it along with the eyes and the face. But this time the eyes and face said something different. The task had changed but the intent remained the same.

As the innocence of childhood flowed between me and Tommy in all its beauty, the voice ascended and descended like a sledgehammer splitting and destroying the happy atmosphere. "You're not a part of our family anyway!" Shock began to set in immediately. Then came the voice of the partnering tongue. "Don't tell him that!" The silence hit me, I felt faint, my head began to spin. The voices echoed in my ears over, and over, and over again. My heart felt the pinch of the knife as it gently pierced my soul. The world collapsed around me. I was blinded and blindsided at the same time. The two voices became one and everything became a blur. "You're not a part of our family anyway…. don't tell him that…you're not, you're not, you're not…don't tell him, don't tell him, don't tell him!" Those words echoed and tortured me for what seemed like a lifetime. Then I could see Mary's face with that look of no concern. She was present, part of the blocking and the memory at the same time. The face of the second voice steadfast in meal prep came forth with force and never giving me so much as a glance of acknowledgement.

There I was, the faceless, voiceless victim turned guilty one. She never looked at me, she never corrected the statement, she never comforted me. My mother, the one who gave birth to me, never even acknowledged me as her son at this pivotal moment of my life. I was simply the object, a byproduct of sorts. As my world crumbled around me, my head feeling light and my vision suddenly blurred, it was decision time. Who is Alvon Davis? My mind began to race. My thoughts were running wild while my emotions were frozen in time. I soon came to a decision. Realizing that I was in this world alone with no family, I decided I had to live with that reality. I had to figure out how I was going to live with this family until I was old enough to move out on my own. I needed a survival plan. I was not a son. I was not a brother. I was an outsider, adopted and brought into this house to live as this Alvon Davis. But I could not live for him anymore or any longer than I absolutely had to. I immediately began to formulate a game plan of separation and escape.

My plan started immediately. My first step was to detach myself from them. I had to learn to live alone because now I knew I was alone. I had no parents, no siblings, no family. If I was going to survive when I was finally old enough to leave, I had to learn to live independently right away. For me this was the end of all relationships in this house no matter how weak or how strong. This meant the end of Alvon and Tommy. At the conclusion of the matter, I would end up losing over 30 years of bonding and relationship with my younger brother because of these words. And years later when we would finally be able to understand and fix this broken bridge, he would die within two years. Eight simple words would destroy a lifetime of happiness and memories. Eight simple words would create a destiny of sorrow, pain, and insecurity. Eight simple words would create a psychological barrier that would prevent me from ever experiencing what it means to have family. Eight simple words would become a mental block telling me never to bring kids into this evil world. But those same eight simple words would create a strength within me that would help me to survive years of pain and anguish at home and later behind the inner walls of the sacred place. Not married with no kids. Hello accusers. Now you know. Judgementalists, now you know. Yes, another story for another book.

"Alvon, and Tommy" was gone forever, never to be revived. This remains the greatest tragedy of my life. Even when we were reunited years later, it was simply too late. It was at dinner in August of 2009 just before my brother married the love of his life that he finally heard the story of what happened to us as kids. It was the three of us that day; Dad, Tommy, and me. We were sitting in the restaurant finally having come back together after all these years of separation. Tommy and Dad kept reminiscing about so many things that happened when we were kids. I can still hear his voice saying, "Remember Alvon." They would laugh and I would join in seconds late as I kind of held my head down. Finally, I couldn't take it anymore. "Remember Alvon" he repeated. "No, no I don't. I don't remember half of what you'll are talking about." I only had vague pictures in my mind that came from the "family" photo album that allowed me to sort together pieces of my life. What they clearly remembered, I only had photos as reference points.

It was time for me to man up and share my experience. It was time for me to tell why Alvon was no more. They sat in silence as I poured my heart out and expressed my tragedy. They couldn't relate and they didn't know what to say. I calmly brushed the residue under the rug to maintain some semblance of happiness in this most joyous season of my brother's life. I bit the bullet, took the back seat, and proceeded as if the past never took place…never to be spoken of again. Tommy's lifelong dreams were coming to pass and that was more important. I was clear on his years of suffering from the separation of our parents when he and I were still kids. He had already lost his older brother (me) and then his parents split up. For him this was devastating. For me it didn't matter because at that time I still thought I was adopted. My brother openly suffered for years hoping and praying that his parents would reunite and that his Daddy would come back. I suffered in silence as I continued to plan for my departure from this fragmented "family".

Having learned to survive without family, I would tell Tommy over and over to stop crying over his dad not being there. I told him he didn't care about us, so it really didn't matter. He had to learn to live without him. But his heart cried out for years, "I want my Daddy." I heard the pain and the sorrow in his voice day after day, year after year. I saw the streams of tears that resulted from a broken heart. But I did not understand why he could not push through. And by nothing less than a miracle we landed on this, his wedding week. The joy in his eyes was unexplainable. Although his parents weren't getting back together, they were back in communication and so was his big brother. To top it off, his biological sister, Rita Edwards, had also entered our lives.

I sat in amazement as we went through that wedding week. Everything Tommy had asked God for was happening. Our parents were reuniting on some level, our relationship was being restored, we now had a sister that offered mutual love. He had finally found the right woman and their separate kids came together as one loving family. Tommy's life was finally coming together after years of challenges yet to be told. His story unfolded to completion in about two years and then he died. It was if God gave him everything he wanted, allowed him time to bask in it, and then said come on home son. December 28, 2011, he texted me. "Happy Birthday." "Thanks" I replied. They are the oldest texts in my phone to this day. December 29, 2011, at about 11am while at work my phone rang. It was my dad. "Tommy died this morning." As he continued with the story, I became lightheaded and almost fainted in the hallway where I had taken the call. I was devastated. I left work immediately and headed home. I was furious with God, and I wanted answers.

I couldn't stop thinking about the years Rodney stole from us and I hated him for it. Then I had to endure Mary at my brother's funeral. I could barely mourn because my head was swimming with the negative things she had said about him over the years. With all the hatefulness she had spewed on him, she had the nerve to sit at his final service with those fake tears looking for sympathy and trying to compete with Rita for our dad's attention. I was upset with my dad because I was not going to allow Mary to attend the service. But that meant a fight with him, so I let it go. Mary and Rodney, look what you took from us. Forgiveness would be the only remedy in dealing with the acceptance of this death. I know Tommy had forgiven them, but I still needed to follow suit. I still hated them both.

As God would have it, I finally had a by chance conversation with Rodney and we were able to settle our differences and find forgiveness. He shared his thought process and took partial responsibility for his actions while using his age and immaturity as his out from full accountability. But this was acceptable to me. Forgiveness was granted and a new relationship started. Although I still find it a little difficult to open up, at least we have a starting point. I don't believe there will ever be reconciliation with Mary for a myriad of reasons. In the continuum of my story and upcoming book perhaps I will go deeper, share more and give some advice on forgiveness, family trauma, and life lessons. It's not always easy to forgive but it is always necessary to forgive. After forgiveness there are other decisions that need to be made that require one to dig deep inside. It is the question of restoration.

Forgiveness is required by God to receive eternal life in heaven. I used to wonder why. Then I thought about what Christ did on the cross. I thought about the literal countless sins that He died for. How can we refuse to forgive the small number of sins perpetrated against us when He took on the sins of the world for all time? This made sense to me. And although it made sense, it was still hard to move into the realm of forgiveness for intentional infractions. It's easy when we know someone did not intentionally hurt us, but when it is intentional it simply is not so easy. This is a growth process, a prayer point, an humbling experience, and a mind changing life essential. While this forgiveness means a one-sided decision to move past a situation, it does necessarily mean restoration.

Restoration is the decision and process that one must go through or engage in after forgiveness is granted. It requires the cooperation of both parties. It is a bilateral act unlike the unilateral act of forgiveness. And while both parties must be willing to reestablish the pre-damaged relationship, forgiveness only requires the absolute action of the injured party. We like to engage in some kind of conversation whereby the offender acknowledges your forgiveness, but it is not essential. To better comprehend the ideology of this concept, we simply engage the fact that there are offenders who are no longer with us. They passed from this life leaving us with the hurt, pain, suffering, and agony of their infractions. We will never hear them say, "I'm sorry." But not hearing those words does not prevent us from saying, "I forgive you." And never being able to engage in conversation that might follow these phrases does not prevent us from offering forgiveness. Thus, we come to the fullness of understanding the ideology that forgiveness is for the injured party. But that forgiveness does not automatically enter the realm of restoration. Restoration is an after-forgiveness decision that acknowledges the freedom of one to forgive, forget, walk away, and proceed in life free of the damage. Hear me, I am a Lion! See my tears. I am a Black Man and I do cry.

With this glimpse into my early childhood, we segway into my teenage to adult years. We enter the realm of religion and spirituality. Maturity and knowledge teach us the difference between the church and ministry. I like to refer to the church as a hospital. As an analogy that would imply that the church is a place where people who are sick go to get healed. It would lead us to believe that the church is a place where love and care would abound as one goes through the process of deliverance and healing. It would cause us to venture and explore the idea of living among brothers and sisters who embrace each other, support each other, and build each other up. Truth be told these are probably the experiences of the vast majority of those entering the hospital. But then there is that small percentage of us that end up in the back offices beyond the sacred place. We find ourselves as part of the hospital staff. And among the staff there exists a separate standard of rules, regulations, and circumstances.

Corporate America can be a dog-eat-dog world full of deceit, destruction by competition with mass usury dressed up as the lies of pursuing the great white hope. But we know the truth. The great white hope, the "American Dream" is only intended for those of a certain hue. That hue is not dark. It is not Black. The psychological and historical truth of this systematic truth should create a culture within the Black Church that fosters all the values, characteristics, and qualities that express pure love, care, and protection for each other. Let us start this journey under the premise that no one is perfect, no place is perfect, and we all make mistakes. And let us journey with the reality that we are all human and that humanity absolutely falls short.

My full experience places me in the minority and yet it is not unique to me. Many have left the church never to return due to something we call "church hurt." I could not wrap my head around why someone who went through some not so pleasant situations at church would leave and never return. I didn't understand how anything at church could cause someone to turn away from God, leave their faith, and desert what they believe in. The stories that I heard just did not make sense. I had some not so pleasant experiences at the very first Black Church that I attended as a teenager. I have a strong personality because of my childhood, so this teenage church experience was a cake walk. Against all their demands, controls, and biblical misteaching, I stood strong. Not having parental protection left me to fend for myself, which I was now used to doing. I didn't know what it was at the time, but my spiritual discernment kept me aware of what wasn't right although I didn't have the actual biblical knowledge.

As a teen it was simple things; fighting with the choir director; taking the kids to unholy activities like swimming and watching movies, not cutting my hair, wearing short sleeve shirts, and ignoring my imposed punishments. In spite of these challenges, I was selected King of the YPWW, and I was being considered for Youth Pastor. Yes, the little tyrant was on the rise in spite of his out of line non-traditional behavior. I believe the Youth Pastor idea was a long shot at reeling me in and thus regaining control of the youth. The fact is, our adult leader and I had complete control of the youth department. Whatever we decided, was a done deal. We were one youth department that stuck together against all odds. And then there was my other partner in crime. The church mother's granddaughter. We were a force to be reckoned with. I can't tell you how many times we took a verbal lashing after church. But we were resilient.

My adult years took on a new realm of challenges in the church. After my teen years in that denomination, I got out. I ventured. I explored. Black and White denominations became my field and walked in them. I finally landed in non-denominationalism. It was here that I got my foundation of spiritual gifts, miracles, signs, and wonders as the bible teaches. It was in this atmosphere that God gave me my foundation. Then my tour of duty began.

Beyond the sanctuary and behind the walls I found myself engulfed in leadership back in the realm of denominationalism. It was here that the term "church hurt" would come to life. Here I would come to understand why others who experienced this dilemma would leave the church never to return. I don't attempt to justify their decisions because leaving God and losing faith is never the solution. But this thing we call church hurt brought me to my knees, destroyed my beliefs, and left me at the lowest spiritual point of my life. It broke me and it brought me to tears. Not once, but over, and over again. Hear me, I am a Lion! See my tears. I am a Black Man and I do cry.

Ministry, the church, and religion can all be life transforming. They can take a person at their lowest point and completely transform their life into something simply amazing. I have seen so many people healed, delivered, set free, ministered to, and developed. The church is the experience of a lifetime when God is the center. It is God who finds us lost and broken and shows who we are in Him. It is God that rescues us from the tragedies of life. It is in God that we find peace and love. God's house is indeed a place of refuge. I will never in any way discredit the house of God nor the man or woman of God. But no man of God, including me, ever loses his humanity. And it is with that understanding we come to enter the realm of the reality of the power of church hurt.

This chapter of my life cannot be fully revealed at present as too many are too close, and I will never participate or be a pawn of the enemy in destroying or casting a shadow of doubt on the beauty of the gathering of the Saints. The bible teaches us that God calls us to different purposes in life. Not just different purposes from one individual to the next, but also different purposes along one's journey in different seasons. So, this chapter is written to those of us who hold the positions in the church that cause people to look up to us. We are the ones that have the most influence to build up, to develop, to encourage, to transform, etc. But we are also the ones that have the most influence and thus ability to bring hurt, pain, and sorrow. How we handle God's people is critical to the spirit of the church, to how parishioners see God, and in many cases how an individual's life is shaped going forward. I'm no angel. In fact, I am guilty of creating a ruckus all in the name of harmony. Fighting the system and standing up for what's right has been my tool of warfare. Taking up arms because of principle is what I did and I always had good intent. But sometimes just keeping your mouth shut is the best solution no matter how well intended. Now that was and is a lesson for me. It's a little something that I'm still working on called, "letting God be God and letting Horace be Horace." Of a truth I tell you, my mouth is my worst enemy.

I say I'm no Angel because I believe that angels always have positive thoughts. I believe that Angels always work under the direction of God knowing the will of God. But me, I can be a hardheaded, self-willed Black man determined to make things right my way and in my opinion. But am I God? Not even close to close. Then there is that part of me that wants to take the real troublemakers and teach them a good ole fashion lesson. But before I act, I think, I reel my thoughts back in and move in the best direction possible. When it boils down to it, everybody thinks I'm a roaring lion. At heart, I'm really a gentle lion. Just seeing people hurt brings me to tears. I just make sure those tears don't flow until I'm by myself. Even the bad guys…I don't want to see them hurt and suffering. It breaks me. And please, when you put this book down, forget this part of the story. I'm not trying to let people know I'm really a softee. I can't ruin my reputation with people running around knowing I have a pillow heart. It's not good for the guy who has to say no and hold feet to the fire.

So, my childhood made me tough. It made me resilient. It prepared me for this part of my journey. And this part of my journey was to suffer this thing called church hurt so that I could help others who are players in this dilemma. This part was for me to feel the pain and to understand why people walk away from church because of this thing. This part was for me to grasp how easily the abused and the abuser can fall prey to this scheme of the enemy to bring damage and division to the Kingdom of God. My message is to the abused and the abuser. My message is to the past victim and the past perpetrator. My message is to the one that might be on the verge of experiencing this horrible fate and to the one who might find oneself comfortable and puffed up with power. My message is to the sons and daughters of the most high God who the enemy seeks to destroy behind the scenes, in the business, in the meetings, in the private conversations, in the planning and development, and in the structural foundation of the church.

When I go to the doctor and it's time for a blood test, the whole atmosphere changes. The laughing and joking stops, the eyes begin to look for needles, and lumps swell up in the throat. Aaahhhh I yell out as the hands begin to tear open white packages. "Mr. Marcell this is only a gauze pad." And so, the war begins. People in the surrounding rooms wondering what the nurse is doing to me until at last the needle punctures the skin. Then the drama is over, the pinch is gone, and I realize once again that it wasn't as bad as I thought. Perception overboard. Had I just let the nurse do her job and let the drawing of blood take its natural course, the drama would not have been necessary. But then what do I do? I walk out giving the same old lecture of "I'm never coming back here again because that nurse tried to kill me." This is in many cases church hurt. But in other cases, it is the body in the street or the surgery in the operating room. Both are real.

I want to make this simple and to the point and from the end to the beginning. If we just remember that God is in control, God sees all, God is with us, and God knows all that we will encounter, then we can avoid this giant of a needle pinch. Small misunderstandings can lead to huge arguments, hurt feelings, and damaged relationships when a little more time is all the situation required. It's like mistaking the gauze pad for the needle. Then there is the issue of not being aware or not paying attention to what's really happening. On both sides of this coin things are often taken out of context. And there are mistakes made on both sides. And I will venture to say that while there are instances where the hurt is intentional, I don't believe that to be the norm. I believe that most church hurt comes from a combination of misunderstanding, the miscommunication, and a lack of openness. I also believe that the misplacement of leadership in the eyes of those being led is a major factor. By misplacement I mean putting leaders in the place of God.

Most of my experience came from internal warfare, leaders fighting to have their way. It is the classic situation of everyone having tunnel vision and no one being willing to "hear" the other side. But leaders are built to deal with the pressures and demands of running a business. And yes, we need to understand that the church is a business. It is God's business. And it has the same or similar aspects of other businesses. There are utilities, rent, mortgage, employees, etc. You get the picture? The higher the level in business, the higher the stakes and the deeper the wounds of war. But in this story my reflection is on the laity. My concern is for those who get caught up in the crossfire and really don't understand what's happening.

In church we are taught to honor our leaders as in the case in any other area of life. We honor government officials, bosses, teachers, etc. Unfortunately, in church, this often translates into us treating our leaders as demigods instead of the amazing human men and women of God that they are. And thus, innocently, we put ourselves in harm's way. We make ourselves believe that our leaders are sinless and incapable of making mistakes. And it is this framework that becomes the breeding ground for this thing called church hurt.

Without disclosing the details of my past, let me indulge you in my mental journey. When my incident took place, I was devastated. I was not devastated because of what happened but because of who was involved in what happened. You see, it wasn't about the incident, it was about the individual. I had put this individual in a place so high in my mind that he was next to God. The revelation and the insight that he grasped from the word was so amazing that I equated it to his natural state of being. It meant that he could do no wrong, he could make no mistake, he could not make an error. And if by some strange reason he did, I could justify it…until it hit me. It took me four long years to recover, to reflect, to discover, to analyze and to understand what happened. Why four years? Because my perception was wrong. I did not have the fullness of where I flawed. This man, my leader, was human. And I was a leader, a key leader. But there is only one God. And I allowed myself to spiritualize humanity in a way that is not intended by God.

Leaders work hard. Many leaders work tirelessly day and night for the good of the whole. Most leaders sacrifice their personal lives, their families and so much more so that they can be all that we need them to be. As a leader, I am there. I spare no expense to help others, to be there for others, to teach others and to see others become all that God has purposed them to be. And leaders deserve so much from us. They deserve our love, our support, our prayers and our finances in fulfilling the vision. But leaders need us to understand that they too are human. They too make mistakes and have flaws and struggles. But leaders put all of their trials and hurts and challenges and shortcomings in a box that stays sealed so they can focus on helping and being there for you. And the second something slips out of their box, we destroy them.

Church hurt doesn't just affect the laity. It affects leaders as well. How many leaders are coming back every single day wearing the smile and the t-shirt with a bleeding heart. To fight the temptation of going deeper, I will wrap up this mental journey and give you some keys. I elevated my leader to a place in my life where he had no business being. So, when he erred, I held him hostage to his mistake, and I became the victim of circumstance. How different would my situation have been had I taken a step back and said, "he's only human, bound to make mistakes."

Here is my advice. Learn to be open to understanding that we are all called by God, and we all have responsibilities to the Kingdom. Our varying titles do come with varying levels of expectations and accountability. As leaders, we ought to be the deepest when it comes to "not only talking the talk but walking the walk...practicing what we preach." We ought to hold ourselves to a higher standard because God has entrusted His people to our care. The time that we spend in the presence of God should be that of sacrifice because of the purpose God has given us. And we should strive to be sensitive to the feelings and the perceptions of those we lead. If we can see us the way that they see us, then perhaps we can gain the sensitivity that is necessary to open the lines of communication in a manner that avoids misunderstandings that lead to damaged souls.

And as followers, if we can maintain in our spirits the fact that our leaders are still human, then we can serve them better. It is imperative that we grasp the fact that with all the spiritual gifts and insight, and charisma, wisdom, and knowledge that God has bestowed on them, they still need our love, care, compassion and understanding. Sometimes we lean on them too much. Sometimes we put them in places that God did not call them to. And they respond in a way that seems healthy because their heart is to simply care for us and that often comes without limitations. Leaders get blinded and blindsided in ways that seem so innocent. But the perceptions, the misunderstandings, the miscommunication, and the misguided purpose of titles creep in and wreak havoc. And the outcome is church hurt.

Whether you are a leader or a worker, we must become aware of how easy things can be taken out of context. We must learn to be open to truly hearing the other side and understanding what is being expressed. Many years ago, I made a decision to believe what I was told and only venture off if and when I actually saw something different. It's called taking people at their word because I want people to take me at mine. I had to learn to open my mind to their reality and accept that in light of and in relation to my reality. On either side, one's reality might not be the absolute truth. But perception is a powerhouse. And when perception and truth are on opposite sides of the fence, you have a real problem. Many times, this fence is where church hurt begins. How that fence gets torn down is where resolution is found. Prayer, supplication, forgiveness, and silence is what I offer. There are some things that we cannot fix. But prayer changes things and all things are possible with God. Remember the power of the tongue. May the spirit of church hurt find its way back to the pits of hell from whence it came and may all who have fallen victim find freedom. May God cause an awakening in your spirit and in your soul that heals every broken place. May the power of the blood of Jesus and the comfort of the Holy Ghost find you and set you free. May you find the fullness of forgiveness and move towards restoration.

Alvon Davis became Horace Wendell Marcell. Horace Wendell Marcell became Minister Marcell, Elder Horace, Pastor Horace, Apostle Marcell, the Prophet of God and so much more (good and bad - another story for another book). But most importantly, the man of God hidden beneath all of these names and titles became a servant at heart with the understanding that life is short, COVID19 was real, and death is crouching at your door. If I ever hurt you, I am sincerely sorry. Whatever you do, don't let my mistake or my wrongdoing keep you from heaven. You don't ever have to speak to or acknowledge me in this life again but forgive me because you deserve the freedom. The power of the tongue is real. Church hurt is real. These powers can alter your life forever. But God has given us power over our lives which includes the tongue. Be free. Be free from every challenge, test or obstacle in life that has tried to tear you down, destroy you and change who you are in Christ Jesus. Today, let the love of God and the power of forgiveness free you from any words that have become haters and blockers in your life. I love you, but God loves you more. Close your eyes, end your journey time with me and let the Holy Spirit minister to you in this very present moment.

The Tears of a Black

ELDER HORACE MARCELL

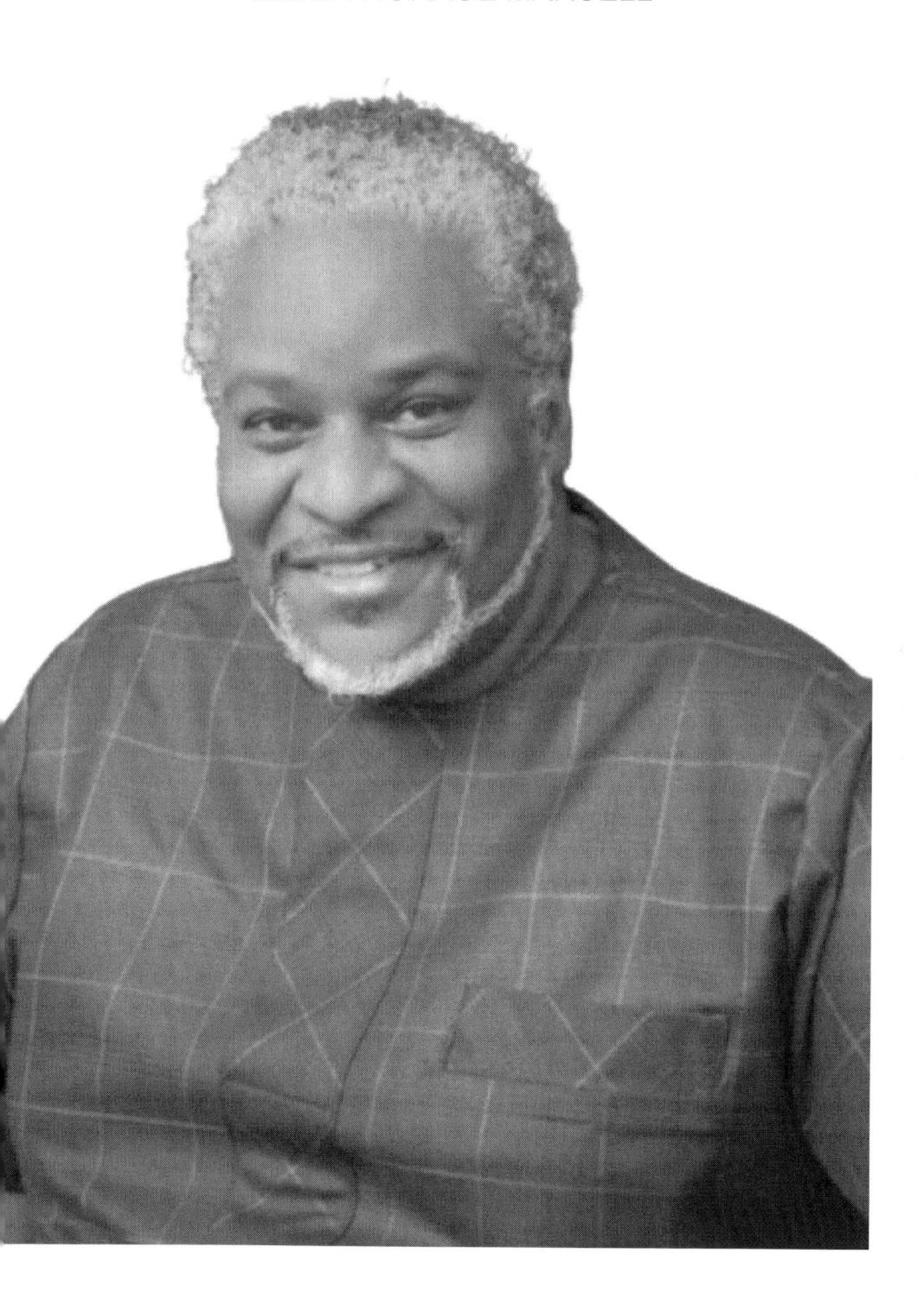

Elder Horace W. Marcell became aware of his calling to preach the Gospel at age 4.

On June 20, 1998, he received his Bachelor of Business Administration from Georgia State University graduating Cum Laude and Local Chapter President of the Future Business Leaders of America National Honors Organization.

He became a licensed Minister on March 16, 2003, under the licensure of Pastor James C. Ward; Antioch Lithonia Baptist Church; Lithonia, GA.

On November 12, 2003, he founded Commissioned Ministries, Inc. tagging the motto "Touching the Nations with the Power of God's Love" attributed to Isaiah 61:1-4.

On March 1, 2006, he received his Prophetic Certification from Life Center Ministries, Inc. Prophetic School under the authority of Pastor Mary Crum.

On May 7, 2006, he received a secondary Ministerial license from the Cathedral of Faith COGIC by Pastor Arthur F. Mosley and subsequently ordained Elder on

June 14, 2014, by Bishop Joseph E. Hogan, Sr., Prelate - North Central Georgia Ecclesiastical Jurisdiction of the Church of God in Christ.

Elder Marcell reached his milestone on July 19, 2019, as he received his Master of Divinity with a concentration in Pastoral Counseling at the Interdenominational Theological Center; Atlanta, GA graduating with Magna Cum Laude.

His Ministry focus is teaching life changing biblical principles and fundamental truths, training ministry leaders in the areas of financial management and church administration and providing staple goods to those in need. His greatest joy is seeing people free and delivered by the power of God.

His mission work expands 5 continents and has touched 16 countries including Malaysia, Sri Lanka, Costa Rica, Jamaica, Ghana, Nigeria, South Africa, Singapore, Thailand, Haiti, Solomon Islands, Barbados and the US.

He is the CFO for Cathedral of Faith COGIC. The financial secretary for Barbados First West Indies Jurisdiction COGIC, the assistant jurisdictional secretary for Barbados First West Indies Jurisdiction COGIC, the AIM financial chairman for North Central GA Jurisdiction COGIC, the finance team member for COGIC National AIM Department of World Missions and the founder of the International Broadcast, "Make It Happen Monday" regular observance in the US, Africa, Malaysia, Barbados and the Caribbean. Elder Marcell is also an actor, having worked on several stage plays and appearances in movies. He is currently a team member with No Nykel n' Production wearing many hats.

His professional career encompasses 30+ years of experience in accounting and finance in city government, small business, sports entertainment, and religion.

The Tears of a Black

CRYING ALL OF MY LIFE

AUTHOR: JEROME 'JWRITEZZ' BRADLEY

CHAPTER TWO

Is there a difference if a boy or man sheds a tear? Some say, "A man shouldn't shed a tear." Many live by this and rob themselves of releasing joy and pain. As for me, crying has no effect on my pride. The storms I have faced in life would cause any man to buckle at his knees.

As babies we cry when we need food, diapers changed or the attention and love from our mothers. But what happens to that boy who does not get that? I went through life with a void in my heart and here is my story.

I was the third child and became the second oldest. Yes, as crazy as it sounds, it's the God honest, truth. At the time, my mother had three children: my oldest sister Tish, my brother Sean, and me. My mother was also addicted heavily to drugs, and she had a tendency to leave her drugs around the house. Sadly, at the age of 5, my brother Sean thought the drugs were candy, ingested them and died. That's how I became the second oldest. I was only two years old when all this occurred, but I do know that's when my internal tears started.

My sister and I were removed from our mother's care and separated. My great grandmother was only able to take in my sister, so I was introduced to the NYC Foster Care System in 1973 at the tender age of two. Now writing this makes me reflect back at how horrible it was to be passed to strangers and not have a family member step in to take me. If I heard of such a tragedy today, I would do everything in my power to be there for my family.

At the age of 8, I was returned to my biological mother, who now had four other children. Since my biological mother enjoyed the drug world, I was left alone for days at a time and quickly learned how to provide for my other siblings and myself. I would steal food from people's homes so that my siblings could eat. Morally, I knew it was it wrong to steal, but seeing my brother on the floor balled up screaming

"I'm hungry", my only option was to feed them any way possible. This was no life for an 8-year-old boy, there were times I wished I was dead.

Traveling on a journey called life, a void that would cause any soul to cry. I would ask myself why. All I wanted was to live a normal life feeling free and safe. GOD had other plans that of course I couldn't understand. As I sit back and reflect on being a young man with no dreams or direction, all I could do was smile to hide the pain and void.

While other kids were out living a normal life, here I was considering suicide. Actually, at the age of 9, I attempted suicide by locking myself in an unplugged refrigerator and was very disappointed that it did not work, so then I ingested roach poison and placed "Neet and Nair" Shaving cream all over my head, in hopes of seeking my mother's attention and sadly she was not around long enough to notice because she was so consumed into the drug life. Drugs had a strong grip on her that she could not fight off.

I would find myself sitting in the window. Calling out to strangers that would pass by in hopes that they were my father. I never met my father and was just reaching out for help, hoping he would come and save me. Those hours sitting at the window felt like days. The emptiness, the pain, the loneliness, the longing for love got the best of me. I lost my purpose but remained in "protection mode" for my siblings. Although I was stuck in my rut, my true instincts were to "safeguard" my siblings as I was the only thing they had. I was all they had, and the truth was they were all I had, and I was never going to let them down.

It pained me to hear my younger brother hollering cause his stomach hurt from not eating. I tried several times to get my mother to pay attention, but it was useless. Finally, someone paid attention and we were removed from my mother's care. While my siblings were running away from the authorities, I was running towards the authorities, thankful that someone heard my plea. At this point, one would think it would be the end to my internal tears, but truth be told, it was a long way from ending.

This time, there were five of us and we were all placed together with a foster family. While I was thankful that my siblings and I were placed together, I still felt alone. Although I was saved, my new environment felt awkward. Yes, we were getting treated much better than we had been, but it was a greater adjustment than I had thought it would be. My siblings were my saving grace, but I still held that void in my heart and I did not know how to move forward. Although I had the support of my foster parents, was provided with a healthy safe environment and all the resources to overcome the trauma I had experienced, it was hard for me to overcome it.

No one understood the anger I held inside of me, I was unable to release it, so it consumed me day by day. I became "a nuisance", a hard to deal with teenager and the quickest way to fix it was to medicate me. Looking back now, I realized that during that period of my life, no one took the time to pay attention to me or try to really break down why I had that behavior. My internal tears poured down more as I grew. I recall at the age of 12, having such an uncontrollable outburst that they had no choice but to take me to the hospital and I was kept for observation. For me, it was a sigh of relief because just maybe someone would take the time to listen enough to understand what I was going through.

There was someone who heard my cries and that was the previous foster mother I was placed with from the age of two to eight, that was Ms. Bradley. She is the one person that heard my tears and fought to get me. Somehow, she found out, I was in the hospital, and she fought to get me back. She came up to visit every chance she could and would tell me she was not going to stop until I was back in her care.

My world changed forever the day we went to court, and instead of Ms. Bradley became my foster mother, then she became my adopted mother. I cried like a baby that day because someone finally took the time to pay attention to me. It felt good to be seen and I started to feel and learn love from Momma Bradley.

Momma Bradley was my saving grace, she took the time that no one else would. The void that I held in my heart for years was slowly disappearing because of Momma Bradley and I was forever thankful for that. Momma Bradley was great, she adopted five other children, who had troubled upbringings. I thought to myself, is this what love looks like. She made that selfless act to adopt us instead of fostering us. Knowing that we were not easy to deal with and all the extra baggage we brought, she was willing to make us her children. We became her Bradley Bunch. Knowing that she did this, when she did not have to, made me want to do better. Her act of kindness gave me life again and I wanted to show my biological siblings and adoptive siblings that in spite of what we have been through, we could still come out of it on top. I remained in "protective mode" for all my siblings, and I took a vow to never change that.

My internal tears slowly disappeared, I began to let down my wall and I invited love back into my heart. I was fortunate to have a biological family as well as an adoptive family and it was my choice to love them all. To be honest, I never got an explanation from my mother as to why she chose drugs over her children, but I did know she deserved her children's love too. She gave me life, made some wrong choices, but still deserved love and I vowed to give her just that.

As time went on, I was able to love people in spite of their shortcomings. I had shortcomings as well and Momma Bradley still loved me. Even with Momma Bradley's love, attention, and guidance, there were still mistakes I would make in order to continue to learn and grow.

At one point in my childhood, I no longer wanted to live because life couldn't be that hard for a child. I was not seen or heard but knew I needed to be the savior for my biological siblings, I made choices at a young age that could have gotten me into serious trouble, but the internal tears and hurt put me into action mode, without adult supervision, I became the adult, but it was because there were other lives at stake.

As a young adult, I looked back on my childhood and said wow, there was a reason my suicide attempts did not work. There was a reason, I did not get into trouble when I was stealing food for my siblings and there was a reason why I was able to live and love again and that reason is GOD.

None of this was easy, you see I felt many times like giving up, but GOD never allowed me to. I did not understand a lot of the things that were happening to me while I was a child, but there was something inside telling me to fight, don't allow these circumstances to define you and for quite some time, it did define me, but then my saving grace came along.

I am not sure why GOD chose that I endure those harsh circumstances as a child with my biological mother, I do believe that in her own way, she was teaching me one of life's toughest lessons; **TO NEVER GIVE UP**. Those internal tears were needed to keep me pushing forward and to only look back as a reference to how far I have come.

Again, some say "men should not shed a tear", but if we don't shed tears external or internal how will we ever learn about life lessons or how to release the pain and love again. As I see it, external or internal tears are equivalent to the circumstances that we endure in life. Believe it or not, it is essential to our wellbeing and growth. If not, we will walk through life depleted and that's no way to live. Imagine walking empty hollow, just drifting and without living life to its full potential.

Internal Tears as a young adult

As comfortable as I was with momma Bradley, I still had my struggles with my identity asking myself who I was? Even though I learned to love again, I still held on to anger and because I wasn't mature enough to know to manage my anger, I resorted to channeling my anger to defend the weak. I saw myself in them;

helpless; empty, alone and yearning for someone to save them. I found purpose in defending those unable to defend themselves. I did not view it as a bad thing, I saw it as justice and never thought about the consequences, but the reality is life has consequences. You can't go around being violated. Fighting became my way of life, but not just to fight, but to get justice for the undefendable. I became their savior. I bullied bullies and made them change their lives. I stood up for many, but one I would never forget was TJ Albert (prodigy from Mob Dep). He and I became friends after I protected him from some bullies. Momma Bradley saw that I was getting into a lot of fights and started to become concerned. She started seeking mental health services for me, but I was rebellious. She thought I needed mental health, but I was too naïve to see benefit in receiving help. Although I made friends, I never shared my whole upbringings with them. I never wanted them to see me any different. The truth is, I was different from them, but I was still capable of loving and being a nice guy to them. I took pride in how people saw me and being loyal to my friends; if I said I was going to do something, I did it and most of the time, it was protecting them.

My "protective mode" has always been my coping mechanism; not to let people know what I am experiencing but always willing and ready to help others. This coping mechanism has been with me from my younger years to my adult years and still plays out. I think I can now refer to it as a quality trait of mine. I saw violence as my means of escaping the void in my soul. If I was out protecting people, then I didn't have time to deal with the man in the mirror.

Turning Point

Whether I viewed my behavior as good or bad, the reality is the consequences caught up to me. I had no choice but to sit and face the man in the mirror. I was no longer that 8-year-old child or young teenager. I could not run and hide behind Momma Bradley. I had to face my consequences. When you are lost with no direction, you can find yourself everywhere but where you need to be. You can run, but you can't hide forever and eventually it will catch up to you. How you handle the consequences will make you or break you. Guess, it didn't break me, because I am here telling my story and that's more than I can say for many.

It was at this turning point of my life that I finally released the years of internal tears and pain that I carried with me longer than I should have. As I sat and faced the man in the mirror (not the boy trying to be the man or the savior to others), I really got to know me and GOD. Surprisingly, I wasn't too bad of a person, just a lot misunderstood. My intentions were always good but somehow demonstrated inappropriately but the best thing is GOD never left my side.

It was during this turning point that I cried the most tears (both internally and externally) because what I was faced with was the biggest thing that I needed but didn't know I needed. It was here, where I found myself between a rock and a hard place and all those that I stood up for were nowhere around except

Momma Bradley and I didn't couldn't understand why. But the truth was, this was my consequence to face, and I would face it as GOD saw fit. At this point, I was no longer angry that no one was there, I even told Momma Bradley not to care or worry about me no more, that I would be just fine. I kept telling myself, this is my consequence, and no one will face it but me. I made the decision that there was no more hiding, I had to step up and finally be the man I needed to be.

Each moment of every day, I reflected on what got me here because in my eyes, I was protecting those that I loved and those that couldn't defend themselves. It was here that I acknowledged that society saw the way I was living as wrong and to be productive in society, one must confirm and follow societal rules. I reflected to my younger years, running the streets for food, asking myself should I have gotten in trouble then, where would my siblings have been, but that was not the time for me to face my consequences cause GOD knew why I was stealing food.

It was also during this time that I discovered GOD's unconditional love for me and my life. HE walked with me through every adversity of my upbringing and especially during my turning point. It was HIS plan on my life, so when I got to my turning point, I was sure not to go back to the old me. He had me endure the internal and external tears, so I would regain my purpose in my turning point. Prior to my turning point, I thought I had no purpose, no direction and was hopeless. It was in my turning point that I realized I always had purpose, direction, and hope, just was not channeling it the inappropriate way. Prior to my turning point, I played protector to my loved one and others, but in my turning point, I accepted GOD as my protector. The one who showed me true unconditional love. How can I not understand that? I survived all that I did because of GOD. HE showed me the greatest gift of life: HIS LOVE and ACCEPTANCE. HE forgave me and for that I needed to forgive myself and I did just that. So how did I move on from my turning point? By never turning back to that negative behavior. GOD allowed me to endure, so I can share myself and my gift with the world. I am a protector because GOD needs me to be not because man wants me to be.

Moving Forward

Can an old dog learn new tricks? Some people get complacent and comfortable in what they do because it is feeding an impulsive need or desire. That is how the devil works to keep the old dog doing the same tricks. Moving forward for me, meant that I rely on GOD to guide my steps, heart, mind, and soul. People wondered if I would survive going back to the same place that I found so much trouble in and were very surprised when they heard of the good, I was doing. I gave back to those same individuals that wanted to see me fail. Many asked how I could give back after all I had done or went through. I would respond; simply because GOD told me I needed to give back in a healthy, positive, and encouraging demeanor. Moving forward meant I only looked back as a point of reference, not as a place I would dwell in. GOD truly covered and saved me. Those internal tears that I shed throughout my life were with purpose although I didn't know it at the time.

In life, we as men, as women, as people and as GOD's children need to know our value and worth, there are obstacles we must face and endure. Some are able to overcome it and live a life full of purpose, grace and love. Some unfortunately cannot. My internal tears made me stronger than I could ever imagine. Accepting GOD's love as the guiding light in my life helped me to continue walking in my purpose. The only opinion that mattered to me was of GOD. Blessed to have found my purpose and use it as GOD sees fit.

So today, When I view myself in the mirror, I cannot help but to get emotional to know where I once was, to the man I am today. I am very proud, and I want you to know that it is NEVER TOO LATE, TO CHANGE. Do not allow FEAR to stagnant or rob you of living instead of existing.

JEROME 'JWRITEZZ' BRADLEY

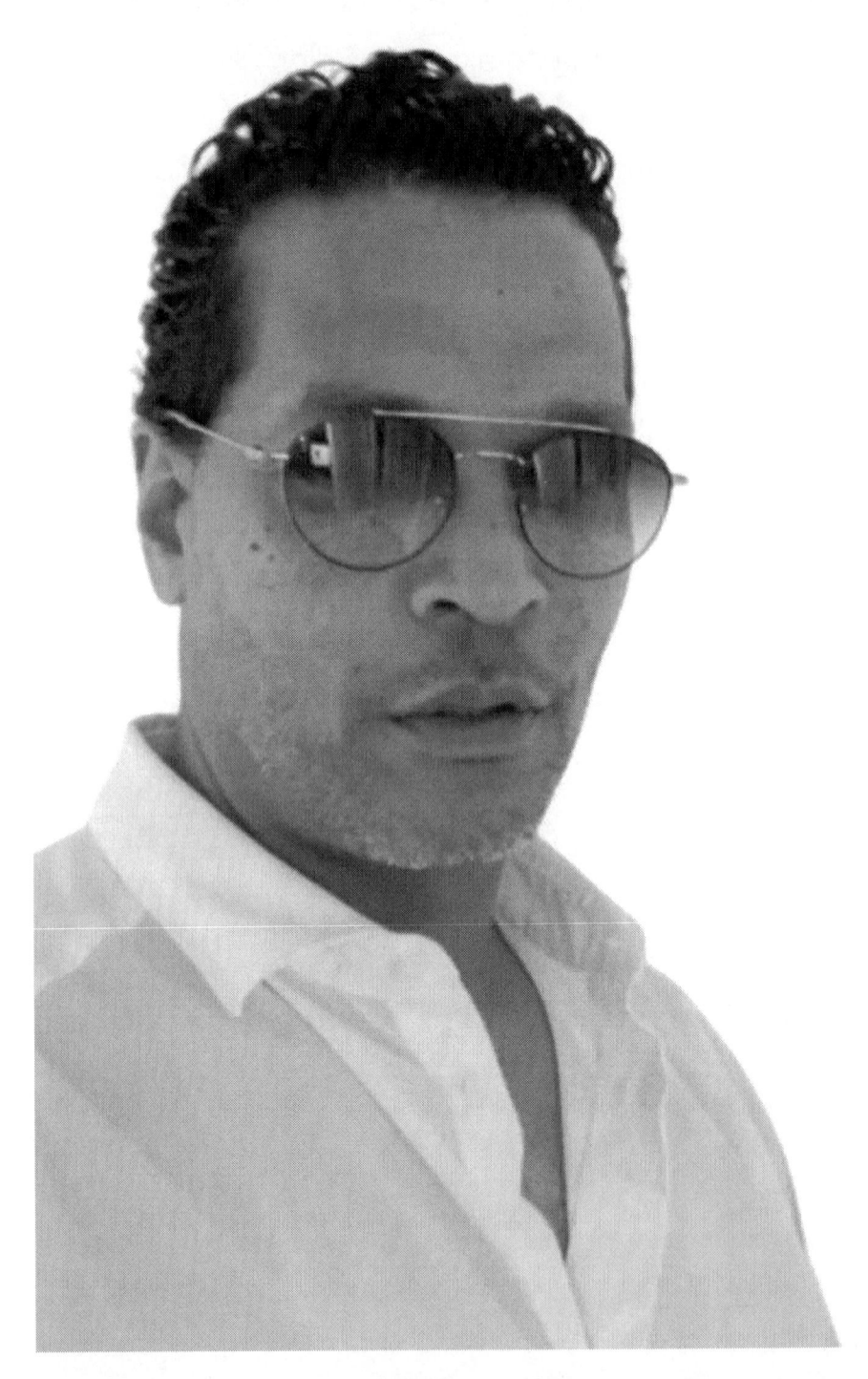

Jerome Bradley was born in Harlem, NYC and raised in Jamaica, Queens NY overcame a lot of adversity, heartache and disappointment from a young age. As he puts it he is "From Hell to Excel". His motto is NEVER GIVE UP and he is truly a walking testimony of that.

Deprived of a real childhood at a young age, Jerome walked through life with a void in his heart and always in "protection mode" Jerome was separated from his biological siblings and family, not once but twice, gained five adoptive siblings and an adoptive family. His story is very unique, sad but encouraging at the same time. He recalls that his strength to fight started at a young age but not only for his survival, but also for the survival of his biological siblings. In the streets at a young age, when people hear that they think selling drugs or robbing, but Jerome was robbing restaurants and trash cans for food to feed his biological siblings, who he recalls were screaming of great hunger, a sound of cry that he never heard before, how could he not help, he thought?

As he puts it, it's not where you been, its where you are headed. He acknowledges his past has shaped him into who he is today, a stronger believer in GOD and recognizes that GOD is the only reason he is HERE TODAY!

Jerome is a lover to all; he feels that everyone has some good in their heart even if they are unable to demonstrate it. His outlook on his own trials, obstacles and life is truly inspiring and motivating to all that he comes in contact with.

Jerome enjoys sharing his life story to uplift, inspire, and motivate others simply through his words, whether it be through his musical poetry, conversations, daily inspirational speeches or most recent through his writing in a book.

Before anything, Jerome is a GODLY man, a family man, a musical poet, performer, writer and motivational speaker and his common theme is to uplift, motivate and encourage others.

The Tears of a Black

Roaming Around Free

AUTHOR: FOREE SHALOM

Roaming Around Free

*Sometimes I wonder what it would sound like
if a lion could really speak?
And would his voice remain a piercing force of energy
that can be heard from wherever he stands?
Would his roar still echo loud and clear?
Or will we be able to recognize the deep down passion
coming straight from his heart?
And how will we determine if it's sincere or not?
Because as far as we all know,
A lion is a symbolic representation of royalty.
His loyalty is a building block of honor,
distinguished by his noble strengths
such as courage, bravery, and power!
He's a strong willed and fearless beast by nature.
He'll never allow you to see his weakness.
He was created to be a natural born leader,
crowned as the king of the jungle,
known to rule with confidence in any given situation.
Truth be told,
he is almost nearly extinct around the world today,
but the soul of this beast will never be complete
without the pride and joy of a royal queen by his side.
The lioness is the key to his survival which he relies on
while roaming around free in a hostile environment.
So, let's explore the journey one is destined to take*

*in order to meet the right mate in the wilderness of America.
It's time to take a walk with me,
"I am a lion!"*
-*Foree*-

CHAPTER THREE

"A black man that can't express himself to a woman is not a genuine man, and a woman that's holding back from taking a good man's hand in marriage probably doesn't deserve a man at all." - Foree -

A true sign of growth in a relationship is not one-sided and too much dead weight on one individual may be a burden. If your partner can't make a balanced investment, you should consider moving on with your life. I'm just speaking my mind and my thoughts could sometimes come off like philosophical poetry. So please forgive me if I say something you don't agree with, but sugarcoating is not a part of my story or vocabulary.

Before we get started, how many black men (Israelites) you know right now willing to share their emotions and feelings in the open? This is a very rare occasion nowadays, especially in this cold world full of concrete hearts. And sometimes we feel like expressing ourselves might make us look vulnerable or soft in the eyes of the next man but walking around playing the hard roll 24/7 is a waste of time if you ask me. As long as I know, I live a life of contentment and my strength is far from being weak. I could care less what other people think but I can only speak for myself. And for that very reason, I never thought it was necessary to convince someone my heart is pure love when my soul is deep enough to make it known. Anybody within my circumference can tell you I have a lionhearted spirit and whoever has a hard time understanding me should start searching for one. It's not in my nature to put on a front for a bunch of heartless people that probably wouldn't send a heartfelt condolence to my family if I pass away today or tomorrow. Besides, "A lion doesn't concern itself with the opinion of sheep." - George R.R. Martin -

Calculating my steps is the only way I learned how to survive. When I stride, my movement can be prudent and gentle at the same time. I have no fear of any challenge ahead of me. Women always say they have a hard time trying to figure me out, maybe that's what they find interesting. But whatever it is, I know it's all love and I don't mind being uniquely different in my own right. My authenticity is unquestionable. For the most part of my life, I did my best to mimic the footsteps of Christ and still do to this day. So, with all praise due, whoever doubts the way God (Allah in Arabic or Elah in Aramaic) created me must be the devil. To simply put it, I feel like I got the swag of a prophet.

Demonstrating my credence has nothing to do with me stroking my own ego. As a black man in America, I just know what I bring to the table and what I'm looking for in a woman. Now let me make something overtly clear before I move any further, "I am not perfect!". And I don't expect her to be perfect either. Endearingly, I desire a queen solely based on her worth and whether she has the qualities of becoming a wife. If this is the class she attends, she'll already know exactly where I'm coming from because it's self-explanatory. Her mind and personality is undoubtedly the truest impression. The way she thinks and speaks is what attracts me, but it's like paradise on earth when her beauty compliments it, that alone is a complete turn on. And speaking from the throne of a king, my queen only needs to portray herself to be confident and perfect enough for me because most of my damage always came from women that allowed their insecurities to do it. A woman with a lack of confidence more than likely will be the one that'll ruin you the most.

"Failure is the mother of success." - Chinese Proverb - My whole life has been a complicated journey of ups and downs, but I still remain optimistic. I find knowledge and wisdom in every step of the way, keenly embracing every one of my flaws and imperfections with all humbleness. Every morning before I step foot out the house, I wake up with a mindset that only God is perfect and worthy of all praise. It takes a bona fide man with a thinking mind to understand and realize this is what makes him human. My actions, purpose, and worship create my image. Very close observation of the prophets and messengers - the best examples of role models that walked the face of this earth - inspired the vision I needed to be successful in this life and the hereafter. The demonstrations they left behind is what keeps me on a straight path. May peace and blessings be upon them all.

Granted this message I wish to convey, may come off as sounding too religious but it's the channel for truth. It's easy to claim you're a good man or woman but can people determine that without you telling them with your own words? And can your overall personality match how you identify yourself? If so, that's when you have to show and prove it. The last time I checked in the biblical scriptures, even Jesus (Isa in Arabic or Yeshua in Aramaic) himself said, "Why do thou call me good? There is none good but one, that's God!" So as far as my character is considered, I do my best to exemplify what it takes to be a gentleman. But please don't take my kindness for weakness because the lion is not always asleep.

However, I could remember from time to time a woman would compliment how fine she thought I was but the voices in my mind were always telling me something completely different. Plagued by uncertainty, there were moments I could hear my self-doubts interfering with my self-assurance. I often thought this low self-esteem resulted from me being young and immature until I learned maturity is not a matter of age but rather a reflection of my personal development. This means that I finally realized experience is the best knowledge, but it took a while to become mature enough to understand my own philosophy. In the past, I probably let a lot of blessings slip away listening to the cunning whispers of Satan. And to call out his motive after falling for his tricks, every time I feel like I meet my match made in heaven, you best believe he's plotting and planning to come steal my joy. And any woman that's unaware of all his deceitful strategies, it'll be a matter of time his manipulation overpowers her in which she is the intended target in the first place, never fails.

In the midst of all my frustrations, at a certain point in my life I started losing hope in finding my queen. I assume in the heat of this moment it was his open opportunity to start attacking me from every direction once my faith became weakened. But each ambush was unsuccessful because the protection from the angels around me helped lift my spirit back up whenever he tried to break me down. I always felt like the victory was still in my favor even when it seemed like I was coming up short. God is the only one that knows what's best, he'll determine when it's the right time for me to settle down again. And there's no better timing than perfect timing, it's already written in the book of life.

Judging by my opinion, I know some people don't believe in the law of attraction but it's very evident in my world. My imagination is always painting pictures that eventually come into existence. I remember one night I woke up praying to God for a woman that could match my mentality and the prayer was answered right away. Miraculously in the matter of weeks, she was standing right in front of me like the queen I had seen in my dreams, and I just knew she was meant to be in my presence from the first time I laid eyes on her. Based on my evaluation, he manifested all the divine signs in plain view on top of her displaying all the qualities of a keeper. Everything felt so right I doubt it was wrong. And if it's such a thing as the opposite version of me, she is unquestionably the one without second-guessing. But God can do what he wills and send it our way as a trial. Now imagine how it feels to be in a position of losing a potential soulmate when she finally arrives.

Keep in mind, I always overcome my struggles but it's not easy being the man I am. As a practicing Muslim (one who submits) in America, my religion (way of life) is always the final factor in my quest for love and marriage. The propaganda and stigma alone will keep people deluded from the facts.

Listen closely, I understand it's hard for a Christian woman to accept the views of a doctrine that's not a part of her upbringing because I come from the same back story. But I never thought my belief would be the reason she decided to take a step back after knowing my stance from the jump which was immensely misleading. I admit, it broke my spirit for a while because I had no idea, she would make a biased decision when it was clear God introduced us for a reason. I was confused in the very beginning because she said it was a period she thought about reverting herself, even mentioning her uncle being a Muslim. She never clarified whether he was a member of the Nation of Islam (NOI) or not for that particular matter, but I don't follow the teachings of the Minister Louis Farrakhan, with all due respect. I study the Sunnah of the prophet Muhammad (PBUH), it's a major difference but that's another whole topic. As a matter of fact, there is no compulsion in the religion of Islam (Submission to the will of God) and I just practice mine accordingly without going to the extreme, this was something I always avoided. I was taught not to cast stones at anybody, so I was never overly biased and still hold on to my core Christian values at the same time. Besides, I just know how to keep that old, new, and last testament mindset because the truth is far from error and it's never up for debate. Belief without reasoning is just like having no belief at all.

Many people fail to realize everything in this life is a test, that's why I know my faith is always being examined day in and day out. It's always challenging but I'm still standing firm regardless. And I know if I continue to delight myself with God, he'll continue to bless me with the desires of my heart. I notice this confirmation every single time he manifests his power by sending me the type of woman I ask for in my prayers. It only makes sense to pray for someone that'll aid me in becoming the best that I can be as a black man in this endangered society, especially when I feel like the whole world is completely against me.

Needless to say, as soon as she started asking me how come I didn't consider finding a Muslim woman to marry, I knew exactly where she was going right then and there. But I just never saw anything wrong with marrying a true Christian woman as long as she was worthy enough. That was just like me asking her, "What was the problem finding a Christian man at church to take your hand in marriage?" A blessing is a blessing, and I learned my lesson from being ungrateful early on in life. That's why I could recognize wife material when I see it today.

On the other hand, I just felt like we had so much more in common than anything. Any honest woman that knows her worth, deserves a husband with the same likeness. Morality is the key to my heart and **the fact she carried herself in a modest way** coming from a society full of moral degradation was enough to open it up.

Piety is the gateway to paradise. A seductive woman that doesn't value herself is scary and I no longer find comfort in sinful pleasure. I'm not interested in a woman that's proud about open sin, knowing it's morally wrong, even though she has a free will to do it. I just refuse to let her demons drag my soul to hell when I'm constantly fighting off my own. So, if it takes me praying five times a day or more in order to seek refuge from the evil whispers of Satan, it is what it is. Queen Mary (Maryam in Arabic and Aramaic), the blessed mother of Jesus, highly respected in all Abrahamic faiths, was undoubtedly one of the purest examples of what it means to be a God-fearing woman walking this earth. For all those with a lack of knowledge or understanding, she is the only woman mentioned by name in the Quran with a whole chapter dedicated to describing her immense piety and devotion. The chastity and faith she displayed alone will never be replaced or questioned. And from this point moving forward, any woman that I meet with similar standards is truly a blessing in my eyes, especially if she keeps herself covered in a humble manner. Sometimes I could still feel my heart aching knowing how close I came in life to marrying someone that reminded me of her character. It was coming to a point I began to question myself, why would God send me a gift like her, then take it right back?

Respectfully speaking, soon after our first disagreement, I immediately noticed how some of her responses were giving off a strange vibe allowing her idea of sanctification to go from a moderate level to being somewhat contentious. But please don't get me wrong, her reputation is still undisputed. When two people love and fear God from different perspectives, I understand it could become a sensitive topic, especially for a woman when her emotions and feelings are involved. And me being an honest man, I deal with more logic and fact, something I have a hard time controlling. But I truly regret that things became difficult for us to move forward when it's already arduous enough to be a productive black man in this country where we were born to go through hell in our search of heaven. So, I never expect a good thing to come easy because the longer it takes to connect with someone extraordinary may more than likely be the one worth holding on to forever.

Sometimes it can be puzzling finding the correct words to make things right and by the time I did it was probably too belated, so I just kept it moving. Reflecting back, I had to take a look in the mirror and remind myself that not only am I losing a good woman but the same woman losing a good man as well, it works both ways. I'm just glad our understanding was reciprocal.

Truthfully, the best part about it, I got a chance to meet my potential wife because I just knew she was out there somewhere. So, despite the fact we decided not to follow through with an engagement, all I can do is wish her the best because I know marriage will eventually introduce itself to me again. In the meantime, I'll just leave my door open just in case she decides to walk back through, only if it's not too late. Wedding rings come in many different sizes and the thoughts of marriage in my mind are still magnetic.

Underneath the surface of it all, I still believe we would've been a good match for each other because we were too much alike not to notice. But we also know two people can't walk together unless they agree. So here I go roaming around free again, at least until another blessing comes my way, even though I feel incomplete starting back over from square one. I'm just glad we found a peaceful resolution in our decision and were able to keep a platonic friendship for a period of time. For some strange reason, my spirit keeps convincing me to check on her more often, but the thought of her ending up in the arms of another man one day is enough to make me keep my distance from being heartbroken.

Very few women I come across can match my discipline. Sometimes I feel like the way I carry myself might be too intimidating for the average woman without it. Besides, as a practicing Muslim, I have to keep reminding myself to avoid contact with random women I find physically attractive. Every interaction should be kept at a modest level, even the slightest handshake can erupt my hormones. My mind is strong, but my flesh is weak, and it'll help me control my desires. According to my beliefs, a man is still considered a stranger to a woman if she's not married to him, and a woman is too valuable to touch if she already has a husband. This is a straightforward and clear sign of respect, only a woman with discipline would already know this herself. That's why I knew she was special; she was paying attention to every detail.

Where do I go from here at this point of my journey or how do I resurrect when society has already crucified my character with different stereotypes?

Sometimes I feel like a lion trapped in a cage and I'm tired of being placed in a box I don't belong in. For instance, a woman once told me I look like a player, in today's terminology, she was basically saying I look like I have a lot of different side pieces. But to her surprise, I started off as a young man raising four children by the same woman from a sixteen-year relationship. I'm not your ordinary man, I take pride in family structure. And just because I'm a Muslim today doesn't mean I want four wives. I can't even take that seriously when I'm out here having the hardest time placing a ring on the finger of one so that's practically impossible for me. I swear by God, "It's like a jungle sometimes it makes me wonder how I keep from going under." - Grandmaster Flash - That's old school. But comparing myself to a lion comes with many different reasons because all men are not considered kings at heart.

Your mind can be your worst enemy. When I was young, I used to think my relationships were meant to last forever until my high school sweetheart proved me wrong. Growing up in a household listening to the oldie but goodies music, the Spinners always used to tell me, "It takes a fool to learn that love doesn't love nobody." By the time I understood what the words to that song meant, the damage was already done, I experienced my first crushing heartbreak and almost cried my poor little self to death. While I'm sitting around listening to love songs, my so-called girlfriend was out there sneaking around. In a relationship, one person's feelings might not always be as strong as the others, and I was a straight sucker for love that didn't know any better. That's when I knew I had to be more careful from that day moving ahead.

Zero is the tolerance level I have for betrayal. And even though I still had to go through a lot of trial and error since then, if you show any sign of betraying me, it's time for me to walk away. I could deal with getting over a broken heart and a few tears, but I can't tolerate being backstabbed by the one I expect to have my back through thick and thin. I remember this wise old man once told me, "A woman could have nine lives like a cat and the only one you'll know about is when you are with her." But this just reminded me of another point I want to make before I tell you how I feel about trusting someone.

Approximately six years prior to the covid pandemic and lockdown restrictions, I was incarcerated for a crime I didn't commit, facing 5 years to life. And it's a well-known fact, whenever a black man's back is up against the wall, he'll make all types of promises and pleas to the Lord in his cry for freedom, especially knowing his innocence. If you beg God and he doesn't show you mercy, who else will? The prison system in the states was designed to destroy us, whether we are guilty or not.

Being behind bars is never easy but after several weeks, all charges were dropped and expunged off my record. Shortly following my release, I came home and met a beautiful queen whom I made plans to marry before having sex - one of the most important promises I made - and I will lie to you not, I felt like the happiest man in the world. We spent over two years in a relationship without being engaged, which should've been the time we got to know each other before taking the next step towards marriage. But unfortunately, I had already broken my promise and fell right back into fornication from the very beginning. I said it before and I'll say it again, my mind is strong, but my flesh is weak. We both gave our power up too fast and it changed everything, but I'll take the blame for crossing the line. I suggested pumping our breaks early on until we got back on the same page, but she started giving me ultimatums when all I wanted was some balance. Sex doesn't keep couples together; we need chemistry, and it was mentally and spiritually draining my energy. Now I had to ask myself, was this love or lust?

Call it what you want, I started becoming depressed and she didn't even realize it. By the time she made a claim of falling deeper in love, my feelings on that note were going in the opposite direction. It used to bring tears to my eyes just thinking about it because I really enjoyed spending time with her, but I became completely unhappy. I felt like she was so focused on her own happiness to a point she forgot about mine. I finally understood no one can truly make my feeling of euphoria elevate without me being in charge of it first because it comes from within. People can only make a contribution to it, but it's also achieved by having a positive connection.

Divorces and breakups are never easy when you care for someone, but my spirit knew it was time to go and it killed me inside because I was right there beside her. For a while, my heart was torn all to pieces and it took me quite some time to recover because I love hard. And I still ask myself until this day, was I wrong for walking away and what was I to do in an unhealthy relationship? I remember she told me to do better in the next one, but I can't love somebody the way they deserve if I'm not at my best. Everybody in a relationship is not happy and everybody single is not sad, I had to learn that the hard way. Love today is unpredictable. It can be blind, strange, and too crazy on another level at the same time. True happiness is about being compatible, feeling alive, energetic, motivated, and not just tolerated. Once I lost the love in myself, I started feeling void. And it's hard for a passionate man that's used to affection not being able to showcase his charm. That's why I'm no longer searching for it, I'll just let it find me when it crosses my path again. Some of us are looking for it in all the wrong places but sometimes a certain place can let a good thing go as well. We just never know.

Furthermore, every challenge or problem we faced was never resolved, they just kept being ignored. Then she opened the door for her family and friends to walk in our business. I never understood why she decided to take advice from loved ones dealing with their own unsuccessful struggles. It's impossible for someone to know what's best for you if it's coming from a place of bitterness. I couldn't believe half of the things I was hearing because everybody was cool in the beginning but now, I got a whole team of relationship experts playing against me. As soon as I started falling back until we could figure things out, she was persuaded to believe I was seeing somebody else. They even convinced her it wouldn't be successful because we had two different faiths and influenced her to start dating other people. A woman that's not in the right frame of thought when using sound judgment will try her hand and she did. After the fact, she put it out there by calling herself making me jealous but that was the wrong move. And how could we reconcile our differences through all the rumors and lies? I did my best to hang in there long enough to compromise but to no avail it never resonated so the relationship was basically coming to its end. I guess she felt like her people had all the answers. Misery is the company of Satan.

Guidance is not accepted by someone that feels like they should have complete control of everything and accepting direction is only meant for those who want to take the best path in life.

Here I am, on the verge of pulling myself out of the middle of an instigated relationship just to find her people spying on my page, claiming I was traveling back and forth out of town to meet other women. Social media is already influenced by a roller coaster of emotions mixed with fake love and real hate as it is, it's a good thing she was never interested in being a part of these trendy platforms. But it was no way possible I could continue dealing with a lot of nonsensical gossip and backbiting on top of fabricated lying by the time she finally came to her senses. Mentally speaking, I said to myself, "drama will always be in your business and wretchedness is not attractive." As an actor, I see enough of this on reality TV shows but I don't plan to be a part of the cast.

Judging by what we call respect, why would she even think it was cool to hang out and accept a late birthday gift from an ex-boyfriend? That's not loyalty and some things are just unacceptable. It felt like she stabbed me in the heart and back at the same time. I was so angry it brought tears to my eyes, and I don't even care to think about it right now. If that was me, it'd be a whole different story. All she had to do was show me the same level of respect I showed her by making the right decision to reject it. But this is what happens when people in the ear of a good woman with bridges that were never burned. I called myself getting over it but it's hard when you feel disrespected all the way around. Now the only choice

I had left hurt me to my heart, and I'm still shocked we let people come split us apart. It was never my intention to cause her any hardship when I decided to take a break. But a power couple is when two people are loyal to each other in a relationship and have a shared vision by supporting each other's dreams, goals, and aspirations. Popularity is created by the confidence they have being on the same page and anything that tries to come in between wouldn't stand a chance but maybe I set my expectations too high.

Knowing how to accept full accountability can carry you a long way because karma is like a shadow and depending on the source of it, it'll always haunt you wherever you go. I don't understand why she wouldn't admit she was wrong but had the audacity to turn around and use reverse psychology placing blame on me without reason. As soon as I saw a pattern, I realized she wasn't capable of holding herself liable for her own actions and never apologized on top of it. That is called being selfish because every one of us is bound to make a mistake at some point but owning up to it is the key, especially if we consider ourselves to be a lock. So let me apologize for whatever wrong I committed. As a matter fact, I'll hold my own self accountable for everything that happened between us.

Lying is a sinful way to avoid telling the truth and if God was to hasten our punishment for it, not a single soul will be left on this earth. A lie is a lie no matter how big or small. I remember she tried to slip one by me in the very beginning and I threw my guards up in a joking manner, but I was dead serious. If I catch you in a small one, I'll automatically assume you'll take a big one to the grave.

Many of us like to say, "trust is everything and without it you have nothing" but I think it's so cliché. If that was the case, why did she break the trust knowingly by being dishonest? Then had a nerve to act with innocence when she was the one that damaged it. At least I was man enough to be openly honest when she was still holding back from telling me about certain things going on in her life before we met. I trusted her with my secrets, knew she would keep it to herself, but she threw it in my face when things turned left. Sharing my deepest secrets was a sign I really planned on being a part of her life but that becomes irrelevant when you can't depend on that person being considered confidant while remaining secretive about her own confidential information. We both have a right to protect our privacy, but I expect you to be as open with me as I am with you. And there's no reason to lie so one of the first things I need to know is, do you consider yourself trustworthy or not?

Now believe it or not, it's almost like we are living in a completely different world today. Times have definitely changed, and people cross lines that shouldn't be crossed. Apparently, a lot of our relationships don't have boundaries where a clear line should be drawn. Anytime a woman converses with an ex or a person of interest without me knowing, she is already cheating. It was already hard for her to trust me off top because she was so used to men fooling around in the past. So why wouldn't she expect me to develop trust issues or how can I keep my trust in someone that doesn't trust me? Opportunistic behavior is now the new wave, and generally speaking, people pay more attention to their own interest over everything so it's hard to determine whether a connection is real or not. And after seeing two good Christian women vanish before my eyes in the past few years, I have to be very careful from this point moving forward. Society has completely changed the way people think which leaves me no other choice to question the person's intentions. Everything is about the benefit of survival now and meeting new people comes with a lot of hidden motives and secrets. I think it's disgusting to see a grown man clinging to an independent woman for his own personal gain without giving anything in return, he should be ashamed of himself for not having it together. Blood sucking leeches like this make real black men look bad. And if a woman outside of marriage depends on a man to give her money for a very small amount of pleasure, it's a form of scandalous prostitution.

Popular belief is now trending with a lot of women looking for the high value man making at least six figures a year from what I used to hear on the late Kevin Samuels podcast. A black man's value is not only in his bank account, but the real value is also what's in his heart. And depending on what culture it is, the definition could mean he's respected, confident, assertive, successful, intelligent, committed, and caring. These are just a few of the qualities which makes him charming and romantically attractive. Normally when a package arrives at your doorstep you expect the full product to be inside and not just a part of it. So, this whole idea of being attracted to his monetary status makes no sense. As soon as we become hypnotized by the physical and tangible things in this worldly life, we lose focus on our spiritual well-being. Materialism is Satan's tool of deception, and we are too busy worshiping money, cars, and clothes, without seeing how deluded we've become by this polluted and materialistic garbage. A lot of black men can show you the money minus the love but a real black man such as myself can deliver the full package.

Queens are the most powerful pieces in a chess game and capable of making all the right moves with a real king behind her. And a confident king can conquer the world with the right motivation by his side as long as she plays her position across the board. We are too grown to play games though, it's time to build. If you want my last name, the foundation starts here. In order for it to stand we need balance, so energy and chemistry is very important. I don't believe in the 50/50 relationship model. It should be 100/100 because only a half of you might hold me back or slow down my growth progress. We both should give our all respectfully and stand on it together. But it's entirely too much enmity between men and women, we spend more time destroying and tearing each other down then building each other up like kings and queens. And they claim it's a gender war going on outside but I'm not participating. I already retreated from going back and forth so please tell me what I need to do to make peace with you on my end? I'm not here to hurt you like the last man, just give me a chance to help heal those wounds he left behind. By the way, somebody lied to you because it's still a fair amount of good black men around, but we are faced with fighting a multi-level war on the verge of being eliminated before it's all over, that's the plan. And after all our blood, sweat, and tears, the last thing we need is for you to help destroy us too.

Remember, "Rome wasn't built in a day." A true king and the right queen can build a kingdom together. If it's solid as a rock, we'll build a palace from pebbles, straight facts. And I'm speaking for the average hard working black man out here, "we are tired!" Some of us are doing everything in our power to build the structure back in our households on top of all the criticism but we need your support instead of being attacked. I feel like the country is manipulating the woman to make the black man look like rubbish anyway.

Systematic propaganda has ruined our lives and raped the minds of our women just to break up our tribes. God created a woman to dwell in peace and tranquility with a man so they both find pleasure in each other. I just hope you realize how important you are to us. We need you to help populate the earth but we out here committing genocide on ourselves with all this division. Without you we can't continue to reproduce. A single woman can't naturally procreate a child by herself. This is becoming a very serious problem, and it wouldn't be a need for doomsday if we don't get it together.

Territory is considered a lion's backyard. I am very overprotective of my family so you can try to enter at your own risk and become prey. As strong black men, we have a much greater responsibility in a relationship which means we should already know our role in a marriage. I was taught the husband is the maintainer of his wife. It's his soul duty to provide, protect and take care of her emotional and physiological needs. He's expected to be the guardian of his family just as well as the wife is expected to be the guardian of the home and children in his absence. These are the comforts that must be met in order to turn his home into a paradise, especially if he wants his wife to act like an angel. Undeniably, men and women both differ in anatomy but are morally and legally equal. A woman can do certain things men cannot, such as having a child in labor, just as well as he is able to do things, she is not sometimes physically capable of doing. Masculine men are attracted by feminine women anyway. It's a reason God gave one more strength over the other, but their bond should always be mutual. This has nothing to do with a man being in control because a woman is still considered equal in her basic rights and human privileges.

Vividly from my perspective, I never considered myself to be the most intelligent person in the room, but I do have a thinking mind which is the house of my spirit. It takes intellect and instinct to find your way in a problematic world. As black men in America, some of us are still hard head and stiff necked to follow instructions. God chose us above all nations to be leaders and gave Moses (Musa in Arabic or Moshe in Hebrew) a list of commandments to understand the criterion of life. It's our fault we breached the contract for not upholding his law and order. Look at us now, completely lost our way wandering around in this wilderness ever since, scattered all over the world trying to figure out why our women don't respect us.

Weighing in by my own admission, a lot of our women have been misled and misguided by the wrong men and I blame myself as well. I remember being in the same boat until I decided to turn back and find myself. I had to think about my purpose for existing, why was I created? Evidently, the one who designed me with a brain to know how to discern and adapt to my surroundings must have all the answers. And Jesus' word led my way to the truth. God driving now, I'm riding shotgun in the passenger seat.

Yielding into the direction of God's divine power showed me how much he is in control. So, if you don't understand my nature as a lion, then you'll never understand where I get the strength to overcome adversity. If I can't lead a woman with the knowledge given to me by God and she provides me with some wisdom in return, we have nothing in common. I need someone who approaches life with an open mind. A queen I could relate to on a conscious and intellectual level. She should be able to think for herself when it's time to make the right decisions because I have no control over her thoughts. If a problem comes between us, we'll know how to solve it or resolve it the right way. There's no need for the stress of an argument, we can just agree to disagree.

After learning self-control is an art of discernment, I avoid reacting to any given conflict without first using logic. Reactions are normally my emotions responding before I have time to think which is often a result of being confrontational when feelings are attached. It's called the PTA strategy; it's learning how to pause and think before you act.

Black beauty is already in a class of its own but this ugly mask we see you hiding behind needs to be removed before it's all said and done. Revealing yourself is an insecure way to get attention. A real king doesn't want his queen on display unless she is sitting humbly beside him on her throne. Somewhere down the line you have to break this cycle instead of degrading yourself in front of society, Satan loves it. I rather see you focus on doing your best at being what the Lord blessed you to do and teach your daughters to be better as a mother. These Americanized standards probably make our cultural ancestors turn over in their graves. A woman that's openly appealing to a good man's eyes may not be to his heart. It's hard not to notice attention-seeking, sexual, and scandalous behavior but real kings will never pursue someone that doesn't deserve to be pursued.

Caring for women will never change in my pursuit of happiness because I know deep inside her soul, she is still beautiful. And despite the fact I'm not completely satisfied with the way I see women act towards us; it still doesn't give me the right to disrespect her. My father raised me well, he taught me to never abuse a woman in any way shape or form and to treat her with kindness. Only a real man with a lion personality knows how to protect a woman without injury or insult. But I'll only show her the same attention she shows me in a respectful manner. That's exactly why I honor, adore, and value her emotions and feelings to the fullest. And even if she never decides to respect me again in return, she should at least return back to her Lord to restore her morals and value.

Dedicating yourself to communication is always a positive vibe, what's understood between two people don't need to be explained again. When it's time to talk like adults we should be able to communicate without feelings interrupting. If we keep the signal between us strong, we can transfer a message that is clear and effective every time we converse.

Every word I have spoken is bound by truth and all we need to do is listen and hear each other out on both ends. A perfect connection is about people expressing themselves while keeping the tone down at the same time and should never place how they feel on hold. If you really have love for someone, you should always be open to having a heart-to-heart talk. How can we get through to each other if we keep ignoring the call? A good way to start is by getting rid of the mood and attitude because immature men and women argue but mature kings and queen's compromise.

Finding the right time to settle a dispute is very important as well but the call is more likely to fail when it's done in the heat of the moment. So, block out all the incoming interferences and remember Satan is always eavesdropping waiting to set another barrier between the connection.

Give me your allegiance so I can marry your soul, I just need your loyalty until the day we grow old. I always remind myself devotion is beyond love, a marriage that lasts decades is when two people devote themselves to each other. Love is just for the moment, but devotion lasts forever. It means a relationship is solid as a mountain that's embedded in earth, and nothing can come between it other than death. But it takes generous support to have a strong partnership. Kings spoil queens and I just need a faithful wife I could treat like one. I picture her being so gorgeous in my mind like she only exists for me and when I look at other women all I see is her face. It's a heavenly sent blessing to meet a woman saving herself for the right man that's willing to wait. And just like I said before, a true engagement according to my belief, is the time it takes to get to know each other before giving up your energy. This will determine if we're ready to move forward so she can leave behind all that emotional baggage she packed up from her last relationship, then it's time to take the next step towards marriage with new luggage. Sometimes I just sit back and think, I came close to getting married twice in the past five years, but I'll never give up on my sister's even if I have to go to the roots of Ethiopia to meet my queen, here I come standing ten toes down on African soil.

"Hurt people hurt people." - Amarillo Globe-Times - I notice your heart was broken and so was mine but it shouldn't give you a reason to hurt me because the love was blind. The look in your eyes alone tells me enough about what's going on inside. And listening to your emotions running rampant like a river, I could understand how you feel. I know it's hard sometimes, but you can't keep pushing me further and further away, blaming me for what the last man did to you. This is not the right mindset because I'll stick by you like a tattoo, all you have to say is I do. It's never my intention to cause any harm because I love everything about you from your head to your feet.

Jesus was a kind man that spoke with passion from his heart. I believe this is something I adopted from the lion of Judah because these are some of the truest words I have ever spoken. Unlike his mother Mary, mine was the first example of what it means to be a strong woman, she was my first love. And each and every one of my past relationships helped shape me into being the man I am today. Whether business or personal, good, or bad, I appreciate learning a lot from every experience I've encountered in one way or another, starting with my children's mother. Credit is well deserved and I'm not ashamed to say, "thank you!" Besides, there's nowhere in the world I should be out here roaming around free, when I know I'm as gentle as a lamb but bold as a lion and don't ever think I'm asleep just because I'm not roaring.

Keep this in mind, life is short, and I just hope you are in it for the long run because I need someone that'll complete my soul to help fix this crack in my heart. Someone who deserves a husband and not just a boyfriend, it's too elementary. Boys prefer to have girlfriends, a strong black man with class is down to wait patiently for a wife but there's no such thing as a commitment without sacrifice.

FOREE SHALOM

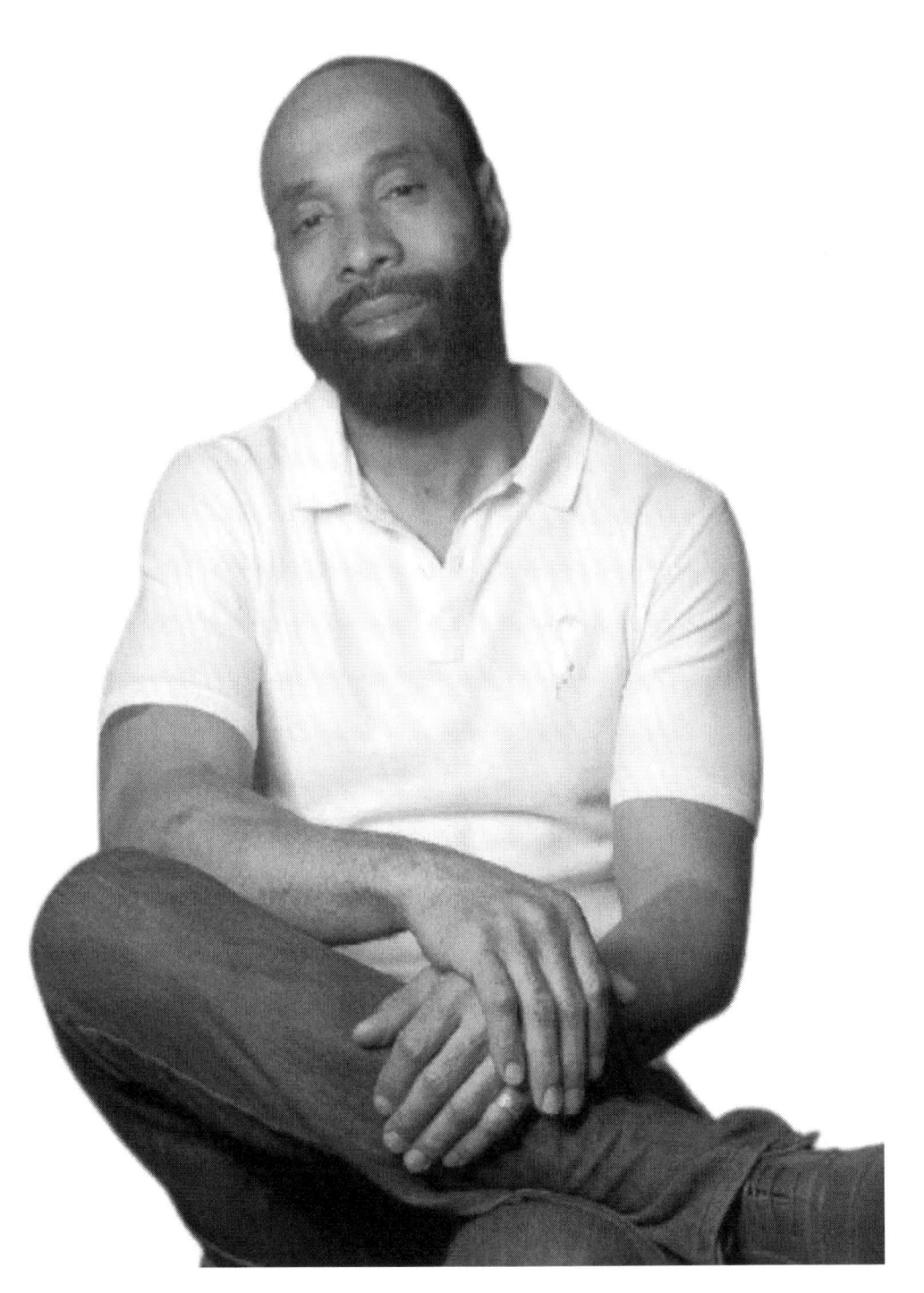

Jerome Arrington, born in Richmond Virginia, professionally known as actor Foree Shalom, is currently a certified Class A CDL driver, and the owner of Green Light Operations LLC. Foree is also an inspiring poet, lyricist, graphic/fashion designer, and CEO of The Poor Family Pride brand, which is an organization aimed to helping the less fortunate. In Foree off time he enjoys exercising, traveling, studying religion, writing music, and recording.

The Tears of a Black

A LITTLE BOY'S VOICE

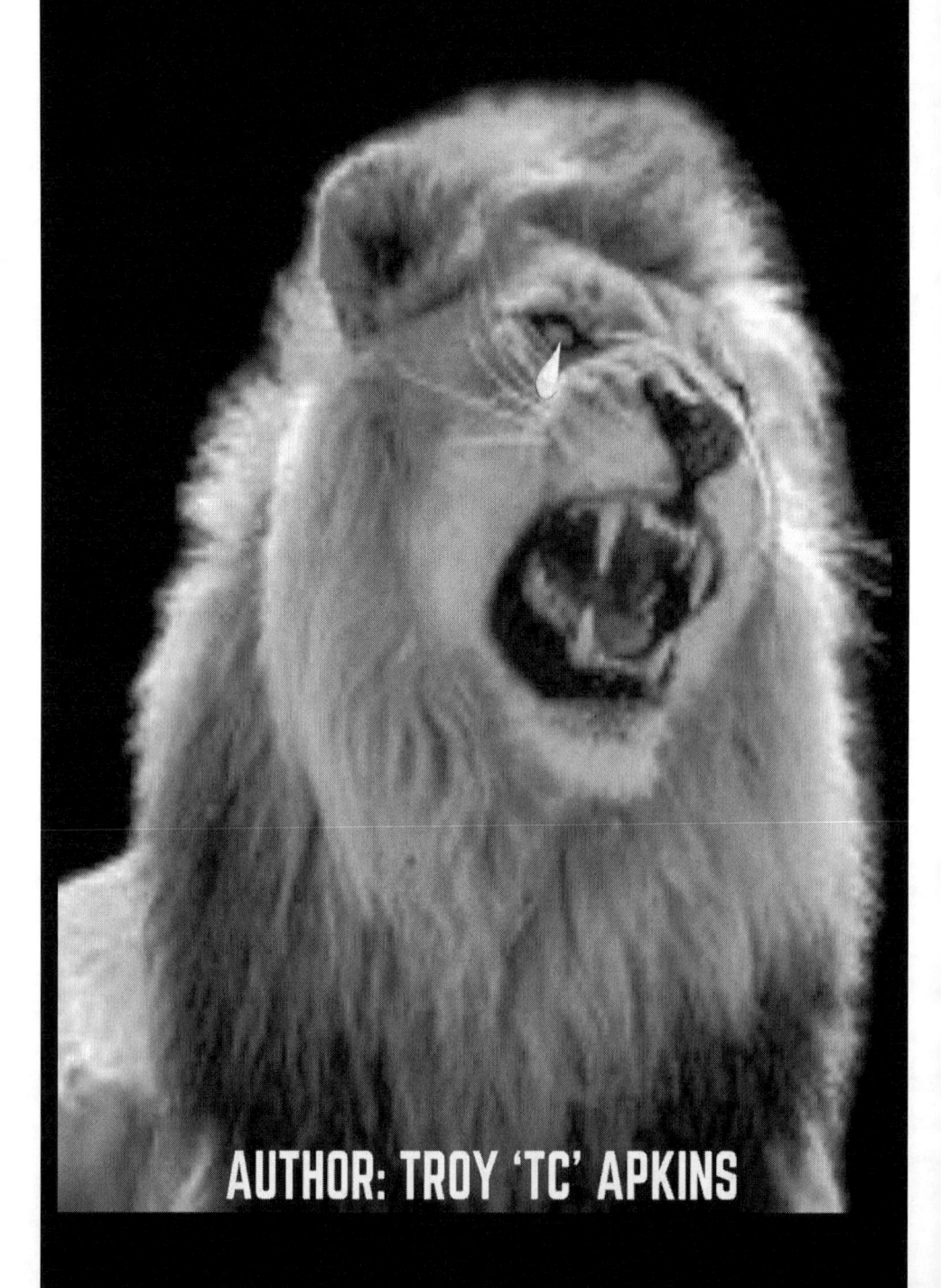

AUTHOR: TROY 'TC' APKINS

CHAPTER FOUR

Let me start with saying that as a child I was rambunctious, full of energy and never afraid to speak my mind. If you know me, I'm sure you would say, I still don't have a problem speaking my mind, but the funny thing is that I had to really search deep for the words to write this chapter.

Until I was five, my life mostly revolved around my mom. Yes, my dad was around most nights. My mom was and is a kind and sweet lady. My father on the other hand was very unpredictable. My father liked to drink a lot and when he drank, he was a different person. Unfortunately, my father would choose alcohol as a companion over my mother. He was a drinker, gambler, and abuser when he was drunk. When my father drank, he would become angry, make outbursts, and keep me in a scared state of mind. He would even raise his hand at my mom. So, it's obvious that by far my mom was the better parent. I found out later that his mother used to beat on him.

So, this is what he knew. This was his method of setting disputes or dealing with his anger. Although my mother was as sweet as she could be to my father, this man would still hit her.

When I was younger, I would watch my father's every move. That's what kids do, watch their parents. When he would visit his friends, they thought him to be the coolest dude. But for me it was all a front and the visits were always too long. I recall once counting to 60 and saying it was time to go after him saying he would be ready in a minute. I was his trophy kid, that he could beg on about being a cool and good father, but he had to forget that I was around him with his abusive language and behavior which was the direct opposite of what his fans saw. My father was a chameleon, charming and lovable outside the house but a totally different person inside the home which was fueled by alcohol most of the time.

My father's friends called him "Rev" for short, a nickname laced with irony because he never was the best influence. Whenever he was drunk, he'd launch into a self-righteous sermon, oblivious to the chaos he created in his drunkard state. It was one wrecked car after another all due to my dad's recklessness. I recall, one morning, the police banged on our door. The police told us that my dad had hit a parked car the night before, wait, that is a hit-and-run, and it earned him a DUI on his driving record. The stench of alcohol on him cemented the charges. My father drinking got him a guest appearance on a local cop show called Blue Lights. The show would record people in certain projects, drinking, smoking weed, doing dope and just being drunk. The cops were not nice at all, and because it was being recorded, they made examples out of a lot of people. And like I said, my father made several of those episodes. It was so embarrassing, and to make matters worse, the kids at school would make fun of me. I even found myself in fights, all because his behavior landed him on Blue Lights.

SIDE BAR: If I had not joined the service, I probably would not be here, and I sure wouldn't be in a healthy mindset. The military took me to places where I learned to release my anger and rage. My MOS would come to be 11B1P, *look it up.*

Again, my father was a bad influence especially when he was drinking. I recall once when my mom went to work the night shift at her job, I caught my dad watching porn and like my father, I rubbed myself, but nothing happened, no milk came out…so I would go to bed. My father was so engaged in his porn that he would forget about me. So, when my mom was at work, my dad was doing porn and so was I. I recall one morning my mom came home early. When she came into my room to kiss me, I was in bed naked, she popped my butt so hard, it burned for days but I had no idea why she popped me or why she was calling me mannish. How was that mannish? I was only imitating my father.

As time went on, my mom said she began to feel trapped, and she felt as if she was being suffocated. For my sake, and for her own, she made a heart-wrenching, life decision. I now know that joining the

Army was her escape, and her chance to build a better life. I was six when she left.

I knew my dad's side of the family but not as well as I would have liked to. I always thought my grandma was well off because she had the open face gold tooth. I eventually got my own open face gold tooth. When my mom dropped me off, the goodbye was brutal for both of us. *Leaving me with relatives I barely knew was a gnawing pain that is still unsettling in my chest.* As my mom drove away, the world spun. I wanted to scream, but the sound wouldn't come out. Part of me resented her for being absent, yet deep down I understood the love behind her sacrifice. And although she made it clear several times to me as to why she had to leave me before dropping me off and I knew that she loved me, I still was angry, and I remember feeling abandoned and lost. To add to my dilemma, I had no idea what was in store for me.

The mental and physical abuse started right away. Soon after the abuse began, I started to pee the bed every night. I figured since I was going to hit anyway, I would give her a reason to hit me. I started wetting the bed at the age of six and it wouldn't stop until about the age of eleven when my mom was able to come back to visit. The visit with my mom was a beacon of hope. One constant comfort throughout my childhood was my mom's advice, "Face it head-on, no matter how tough." It's a motto I still hold dear. Something that makes me smile when I think about it was when I was young, my mom would always say, "Chew it up good. Chew it good no matter what. Till this day I still chew anything I put in my mouth, even ice cream.

Side Bar: Funny story about the first time I gave oral, I almost chewed off her *(cookies)*, but that's another book. Oh yeah if you are wondering I have gotten alot better.

Being so young, and not able to defend myself at home, I got into a lot of trouble in school, constantly embroiled in fights. A misguided protector, I only beat up the bad kids like really bad. This culminated in expulsion by second grade which caused my grandma to move us to a cramped, rundown house in rural Alabama in order for me to go to school and to get a new start. The house was not in the best condition. For us to have a large family, it is amazing how we lived under those conditions. To survive, you had to be tough. Throughout the years a lot of work and money went into expanding and making it livable. Despite the hardship, it was still a fresh start. Over time, the house became a more bearable place to live, even though my grandma's abuse continued. I recalled the family whispering about me. I would overhear relatives advising my grandma to be more patient and understanding with me. My grandmother's sisters would say, "Cut him some slack, he misses his mother," but she would ignore the advice. My grandmother's physical punishment would continue when they weren't around. There was no rhyme or reason to her abuse, just a constant pressure to "do it right the first time," oddly enough this principle proved to be beneficial to me later in the military.

She had no problem waking me up to a whipping if she wasn't happy with something I had done that day or night. I wish I could tell you what her triggers were, but I can't. Sometimes it was because I did something incorrect, other times she needed to release her anger. Her weapon of choice was an extinction card, even with clothes on, those cords still pierced the flesh. She would be calling me out of my name. The abuse that I remembered most was one time she dislocated my shoulder, and I had several blackeyes. She would always lie to people about what happened to me. She would blame it on sports or me being clumsy. And if the physical abuse wasn't enough, she would mentally abuse me. She loved to compare me to my male cousins. Granted they were all smart and talented but so was I in my own right, and in some cases I was better if not just as equal. But honestly, there shouldn't be this kind of talk amongst family but that's what poison does. It brings division between people. I remember telling her one time that she should be more like my aunties when she started in on me of how much better my cousins were than me. This mouth of mine wrote a check that my butt couldn't catch. I damn near got jumped when we got to the house. I couldn't get out of the van fast enough before she would take out her anger on me. Although my punishment was unspeakable, it was worth it to tell her how I felt.

I learned the hard way that she did not like to be corrected. One day I exploited that, and boy was it worth it. She had this thing for trying to make me feel dumb. She would always say, "I can't *learn* you nothing." So, in English class I learned that "I can't learn you nothing" is improper grammar. The correct wording is, "I cannot teach you anything." I was excited and amp to come home to tell her that she was speaking improper English. I couldn't wait for her to say, "I can't learn you nothing". Once she said that, I was going to say, "You right you can't *learn* me nothing, you are supposed to *teach* me." You could guess how that turned out. She put a number on me, and yet again, it was so worth it, although the spatula she hit me with left a mark like a tattoo on the side of my face.

Despite the harsh environment, there was a sense of normalcy, no matter how artificial it was. I can recall the charade of family photos. Every few years, we'd dress up for pictures, a forced display of happiness that masked our true reality. The photos with black eyes were a constant reminder of the dissonance between the image and the truth. To seem like a normal family, she had this thing for Ollan Mills. Boy did I hate those fake pictures.

Side Bar: My childhood experiences have undoubtedly shaped me as an adult. When someone promises to cherish and take care of you but beats and demeans you can mess with your mental state. The things I went through and experienced as a kid have affected my adulthood in so many variable ways, both negative and positive. As much as I am working on it, I do have trust issues. I am sometimes easily excited by the smallest thing. I do not expect anyone to give me anything, but the thought of it is a pleasant one. It does something inside me when a person thinks of me or does something for no reason at all for me. The mere act of someone showing up, being reliable, is a gift I deeply cherish. It's a stark contrast to the broken promises of my past, a past that taught me resilience even in the face of disappointment. It releases a sense of hope in me, that definitely stems from my childhood of not giving up even in the midst of darkness. My darkness was the assumption that the people I am related to, wanted to be related to me and would naturally love me. My hope was that one day, someday, maybe one day, they would love and treat me as such. Unfortunately, that didn't happen for me. My mom always loved me, but distant love was not enough to stand up to the hurt my grandmother bestowed upon me.

I wish I knew the proper words to help you understand my painful childhood journey. Maybe there aren't any. Nevertheless, as unbelievable as it is, my grandma would treat me like a stray cat, but she claimed that she wanted me to be there, the nerve of me for being me. Looking back, I realize that my grandma needed counseling for her past. I don't know why she was the way she was toward me, but it wasn't for me to figure that out. I was her grandson, and her job was to protect, provide, and love me, but she failed. Instead of love, I endured manipulation, where she was supposed to provide comfort to me, she chose to treat me coldly. I'm going to be honest enough to say that what I endured left me scared.

As an adult, I've learned to detach from emotional manipulation, a skill that served me well in the military. The downside is that it can come across as insensitive. I crave genuine connection, but sometimes my defenses get in the way. All I've been through; I believe I'm a good person with a lot to offer. I have a strong sense of compassion and honesty. As a man I would laugh with the confidence of a bear when my grandma would bark an order to me. As a man I could finally protect that little boy.

The problem with protecting that little boy was that it caused me to make a lot of mistakes because of unresolved issues and unhealing. My ex-wife, my partners know that if ruffled I could be a heartless, firecracker, in the middle of a conversation or disagreement. I have been working on my emotional connection because as a child I detached emotionally in order for me to cope with the pain that I was enduring. So as an adult I am unaffected by tears. I can detach emotionally if, and when necessary, it may sound hard, but it actually made me a great soldier.

When I look back, I sabotaged a few of my own relationships. I went into my relationships with the underlying mental assumption that I must protect myself from my grandma's abuse. So, when my partners made a mistake or what I deemed to be a mistake or what I viewed as a sign of attack towards me, I went over the top to protect me. In most cases it wasn't so much of what they did, as it was me reacting to my childhood trauma. I'm thankful that I was able to see these flaws and work on them so that I could be a better person and partner. So yes, I messed up some relationships and I have been drawn to toxic people, but I have grown, and my joy outweighs my pain, and my attraction is no longer to toxic people. With that said, at the end of the day, I'd like to think that I am a great guy, with a list of character flaws. But I also have positive character traits that allow me to stand out. What are they you may ask? Well, I'll be happy to share some of them with you. I have a huge heart full of compassion, I am a gentleman, I absolutely love to help deserving people and I just love to make people smile. In fact, I have been recognized and voted ATL's Hottest Gentleman, several years in a row. So, it's not just me saying it but the people agree.

Now with all of my tooting, I must admit that I have a knack for being brutally honest. My childhood has made me a complex man. I have learned that sometimes, I have to be mindful to take other people's feelings into consideration when asked my opinion. In the past, there was no sugar coating it. I used to think that, hey, life didn't sugar coat anything for me, so I'm just gonna give it to you *(whomever you would be)* just the way it was given to me, raw and uncut.

I want to share with you how the relationship continued with my father by sharing a memory.

In my young dating season, I, probably like a lot of youngins, was made to go to church and choir rehearsal. One day I decided not to go to choir rehearsal. Feeling a little frisky I invited my girlfriend over. One of my girlfriend's older sisters said that she couldn't leave unless I brought her a pack of Newport and a Bud beer. My guess was she didn't think I could get the items because I was underage. Fortunately for me that was the same brand my dad liked, and the corner store was where my dad frequented a lot. So, after pleading and lying to the lady at the register that my dad was drunk and sent me for the items, she finally gave in and walked out of the store, feeling good because I had completed my mission. Although I knew my dad would eventually find out, at the time, I didn't care, my hormones were leading the way.

When we got to my home and to my bedroom, we started our porn star performance when low and behold, guess who came storming in the house and startled us? It was my dad, so I quickly got dressed, and ran out the room yelling to tell him he had to go because grandma didn't want him in the house. A week before, he got drunk and began talking disrespectfully to my grandma, so she had hit him with the broom, chasing him out the house and yelling that he was no longer welcome inside the house. He was not allowed inside. *It was like she had grounded him to the outside.*

He had to use the bathroom, which was across from my room but instead of going to the bathroom, he made a B-line into my room. I yelled for him to stay his ass out of my room. Yes, I cussed at my father, that is how much respect I had for him. Nevertheless, as I chased behind him afraid of what he may see, I was relieved to see that my girlfriend was sitting on my bed fully dressed. So instead of telling us to go into the living room or even ordering us out of the house, because a blind man could see what was about to happen. He demanded $10 dollars from me. So, I gave him my $10 roll of quarters I saved from pitching quarters. He knew I had money, he just didn't know where I hid it, so I gave it to him to get rid of him.

So that was our relationship, you would think he would've taken the time to talk with me about *'the birds and the bees'* opposed to paying him off. I am not blaming him for my choices in life, but I am blaming him for the lack of preparation for life choices. Just think of how much better life could've been or my view on life had he played the position he was given as a father. I often wonder how our relationship could've turned out had it not been for his troublesome toxic behavior, blackout drunk episodes, unlucky gambling, or drug use. I can only imagine how close we could have been. Oh well, too bad for him.

I remembered the night before I left for basic training. My dad's sister hosted a going away party at her house for me. Things were going great; everyone was having a blast. Guess who showed up drunk as usual? Yep, my dad, showing his ass and being disrespectful, talking shit about me and to me in front of everyone. My aunt asked me to take him home before he got more out of hand. Really? I told my auntie that it wasn't going to happen. I loved my aunt, but I had to take a stand for myself, and I was not going to allow myself to be abused on my last day before embarking on my new life, but she insisted. So much for standing up for myself, needless to say that my party ended a lot sooner than I wanted it to. My plan was to drop my girl off then drop him off and head back out to see her. But he talked so much shit on the way to drop her off that I was overly pissed by the time we made it home. To make matters worse he didn't want to get out of the car when we got to the house. *Even as I write this, it irritates me.* At this time my grandma had converted the old storage house into a decent living space for my dad, so she could keep an eye out for him. When he finally got out of the car, I went into the house. I assumed he would go to his quarters, but not so, he came into the main house running his mouth so much that we got into a yelling match. My grandma shut us both down. Not wanting my night to be a complete bust, I was preparing to leave to be with my girlfriend and I told my father that he needed to be gone when I got back. As I headed to my room to get some things, he decided to push me into my door as I was unlocking it. He made it clear that he wanted to fight. *Again, as I write this it is uncomfortable.* I couldn't believe that my father was so envious of his son that he would want to fight me. At this point, I had made up my mind that all of the hurt he bestowed on me and my mother, all of the hurt my grandmother bestowed upon me and the fact that he ruined my going away party, he was going to endure. So, once I got my door open, I snatched his ass inside and I started whipping on him real good. I remembered that I had his head in a scissor lock with his head between the wall and the bed. I didn't realize, but I must have shut the door. My grandma opened the door, I immediately started yelling for her to get him. She made my father get out of the house.

This next statement may not be so kind to read but it's my truth. After all the times my father would hit the soft spot on my head, all the times he talked about my mom to my face and to others, all the times he put hands on her, for every time he stole from me, or extorted me, over beat me to appease his mother, not only did I feel like he had that coming, I enjoyed that high for a very long time. Does that make me a bad person? I think it makes me a person that felt vindicated although, I am not condoning violence as the answer. I am just sharing my truth.

Whenever I would visit home from the military, my father would keep his distance from me. I guess because he realized that I was no longer that helpless little boy that he could victimize or maybe he remembered that butt kicking *(I know that wasn't nice)*. One visit he said that someone from the corner store told him to never assault me again. He went on to say that he kept my secret of getting beer and cigarettes in his name, from my grandmother since she thought I was so perfect. I humbly told him I appreciated it. That was pretty cool of him, to not tell my grandmother. He asked me if I felt like a man now. My response was that I was a man long before my time, thanks to him. Yeah, that was our relationship. One man realizing he could no longer traumatize a little boy and not a father planting seeds or wisdom to his son.

He had another son I never really liked growing up. Mainly because my dad would take my gifts and things. give it to my half-brother. Nothing came in or out of the house without my grandmother knowing. So, I'm sure she knew what my dad was doing, I am sure that she was behind a lot of the things he would take. He took from me to make himself look in his son's eyes. I had so much animosity towards my brother for that. I realize now as a mature, healing adult that It was never his fault, he was just a child, a victim of my father's foolishness. My dad took things like my guitars and drum sets, even small little things that had sentimental value to me and that he did not pay for and handed them to my brother. Boy, did that make me really dislike my brother. Just like a contiguous disease, I picked up my brother, like my dad picked on me.

I remember one visit from the military. I was probably about twenty, he was like eighteen at the time, we grabbed some drinks and just rode around the different neighborhoods. We talked for hours when I decided to come clean to him about why I treated him so bad as a kid. Why I was such a jerk when we were younger. I apologized for passing my anger off on to him. He opened up about his issues with our dad as well. We laughed at some things and we truly bonded that night. Isn't it mind-blowing how the man that tried to draw division between us actually bonded us together. Till this day we are still close brothers. Thanks dad.

When my dad actually passed away, people, friends and family kept asking if I was alright because I was pretty numb to it all. I remember me being upset he didn't pass two weeks earlier when the army sent me home to see him. As selfish as that may sound, that is how I felt, and I was irritated with him because of that or was it because now that he was dead, we would never ever have the opportunity to somehow really embrace a true healthy father son relationship.

Nevertheless, I don't hold that hatred and anger anymore. In life you learn, and my father did a good job at teaching me what not to be. Thanks dad.

I had to get to a point in my life, where I wanted better for myself. I had to forgive the people in my life that hurt or wronged me, both dead and alive. Once I came to that realization it wasn't easy, but it was necessary for my happiness. So, I made a choice to begin to live a healthier, and positive life. To make that happen, one of the things I chose to do was try to understand my grandma.

Born in the early thirties, in the midst of the great depression, she was first born. My grandma had to be strong and tough growing up with eighteen siblings. She had nine brothers and eight sisters. Also, she had three of her own kids rather young. Let them tell it, I had it easy. Of course, I could never see how they could say that being that I was abused most of my childhood. Now that I am older, I could understand why they would say that because times have changed a lot since their time, and somehow, they didn't see my trauma.

I have to honestly say she did raise them well. They all went on to be successful, but one died in the military. They live under the village umbrella. Some families would send their children to be punished by some of my older male cousins. Now these two cousins, I'm referring to, were nuts. I mean crazy in the head nuts, both of them. I will share a story to help you understand why I am saying this.

I remember one time as a child, there was a very big Doberman and her puppies and somehow, they got under the house. This was before grandma upgraded the house and boarded up the bottom of the house. Well at night you could hear them so clearly whining and bumping the plumbing. My grandmother wanted my two older cousins and I to go get the puppies from under the house while the momma dog was away. That was a bad idea; when came she chased my cousin all around the corner. So, my grandma called animal control. They came and found the momma dog in the neighborhood and took her away, but they didn't come for the puppies. Since my grandma wasn't going to spend another night with those whining puppies, she had us get them from under the house. Since I was the smaller cousin. I was sent under the house to toss them out to my cousin who was holding a potato bag and putting them inside. I believe it was like five of them total, they were so small and whining for their mom. My grandma told us to put them into the ditch drain. Wait? What? I couldn't believe my ears and I never thought that was cool, but I knew what would happen if I dared to object. The reason why I say my cousins were nuts, is because it didn't seem to bother them at all. In fact, one wanted to stay until the bag went under. YES, NUTS! Nevertheless, they both joined the Army, and both would often write to my grandma, thanking her for being so hard on them and how they would not have made it as far as they did if it wasn't for her. One went on to become a drill sergeant.

That may have been what they needed but I didn't need the hostile upbringing. I used to like my cousins except when they would jump me and pull a wrestling move on me. They would say that I needed to get tough while they had me in a choke hold until I'd damn near pass out. They would punch me trying to make me cry. Boy did I want to kill them in those days. They were my bullies, but since they graduated a couple years before me and a year apart, they had paved the way to where I knew a lot of upperclassmen, mostly girls. I loved my freshman year. For that I didn't want to kill them. So that was the type of family I came up in, it was violent, that is how they communicated, with their hands and always on attack mode. So, with that understanding it kinda helped me to understand my grandma. Maybe she didn't think she was doing anything wrong. I don't know, but what I do know is that I had to forgive. The forgiveness was her lack of knowledge on using other tactics to raise me.

Side Bar: One thing about me that I love to do is to grill. I believe that is something I got from my dad because he loved to grill. When I was married, I would grill every Sunday. I grill now whenever I can.

I'm told that grilling and baking is way healthier. My dad taught me how to pour salt on my eggs when boiling them. So that the shell would come off easy. A nice trick that I still use today. Well, look-a-there, he did teach me some positive things. Thanks dad.

All of my grandma's siblings were very light-skinned. She was the lightest. My dad and I were darker in complexion, more like a caramel brown. So, when my grandma would address me or my dad, she would call us *nigga* most of the time. Black nigga, dumb nigga, stupid nigga, yup, we were some type of negative niggas. She was hard on me but harder on my granddad. Oh yes, my grandma had a husband. He was not my biological granddad, but you wouldn't know it. He was a special man. Let me say this, there is no way I could have lived like he did with my grandma for as long as he did, just no way. He would work his butt off only to give his entire check to her. She would get mad if he cashed his check without her. I never understood that. She would count his hours to make sure he was at work. She would give him an allowance out of his own money, which was not enough to do anything with. She didn't like him drinking, so he would have to make a decision. Cigarette money for a couple weeks or buy liquor and being that he was more of a smoker, cigarettes it was. My grandma would make his lunch most mornings but not if she was mad at him, he was on his own to get to work and fend for himself, yup, she was cruel just like that.

Granddad's family lived not too far from us, just a few blocks away but she would get mad if he went to visit his family. She led her side of the family to believing that my granddad's side of the family were nasty drunks, his dad, brothers, and their lady friends, and was so far from the truth. I remembered walking to the neighborhood park one day and I saw my grandad over his family's house. So, I shot over to say hi to everyone and as always, they were just as nice as they could be to me. I always felt like they felt sorry for me. I could understand, considering what their brother was going through with grandma, his wife. I overheard someone saying that grandma had a spell on him, that he had changed and that he wasn't himself since he married my grandma. They strongly felt this way and had no problem expressing their feelings in the street. He was a great guy to me, although he was not very educated, but he was a super strong man. He was a black man; he was a provider for her kids as well for me. He was really-street smart and people friendly. He was strong and gentle at the same time. He always carried a pocketknife with a cool wooden handle. He would use that knife for everything. He would eat raw onions, just pull out his knife and cut it into another layer. He would be crying, eyes just watering while he'd be just chomping down. We would go fishing, and I could ask him anything. He'd use his pocketknife to cut bait or whatever else he'd need to use it for. I even saw him on several occasions under the carport seating on the stairs, cutting out dead skin from his hands and feet. I cannot say that I'd ever seen him clean it, but I'm sure he did, at least I hope he did. My dad and his siblings had a level of real respect for my granddad. He had been in their lives since my aunt was seven. He stepped up and took care of three kids that weren't even his kids. You would think my grandma would've been a little more respectful and grateful.

Over time my granddad started to develop strange pains. No one really knew what was going on with him and he didn't do doctors. This next statement is the truth, and some may be extremely upsetting to read but the truth doesn't always make you happy. To my dismay, I witnessed my grandma adding something to his meals on multiple occasions. I didn't know what it was, but something in me was saying it seemed wrong and I needed to say something. Remember, I said I have always been brutally honest. So, I told granddad of what I saw and of my suspicions. He initially doubted me, but he eventually acknowledged it was a possibility that what I saw was what I thought it may be. My granddad stopped eating my grandma's food and what do you know, his health improved. He simply told her he stopped eating her cooking, claiming it tasted off. After he regained his strength, he confronted her. Of course, my grandma denied it and fortunately for me, granddad protected me, and never exposed me as his source. I later learned that she'd dabbled in Hoodoo, a practice involving powders and liquids. The realization that she might have tried to harm him, yet he forgave her, left me deeply confused. However, it did lend credibility to his family's claim about her. This experience undoubtedly contributed to my trust issues. I still have a problem with trusting people. People only allow you to see what they want you to see. Some people thought my grandma was such a sweetheart, no one saw that side of her that if crossed or she just wanted to mess with, she would find a way to have people evicted to getting arrested. She knew people back then Mobile and Prichard and by that time most of her classmates were local politicians or deputy sheriffs in the county and surrounding counties. She knew judges mostly from my understanding my dad had a lot of run-ins with. I believe it was something to it because my dad would never be in jail long. I think it's safe to say somehow, my grandma was connected.

I did not find out until I was about twenty-one, that my granddad and grandma had been divorced for over nineteen years. None of us knew, but he stayed with my grandma and took care of her children and me. This man that was not my biological grandfather, was more of a father to me then my real dad ever was. He was an amazing man, and I would think his reward was that he outlived my grandma.

I remember when I was seventeen years old. my high school girlfriend became pregnant, my grandma intervened. To this day, she claims the girl miscarried, but I suspect she may have been involved in some kind of financial settlement for the baby not to make it. Witnessing such events at a young age undoubtedly shaped my thinking. My girlfriend never said anything different, but I did notice her and her sisters, all of a sudden fashion and hair styles were leveled up. My grandma wouldn't bash her like she would normally do. Some things you tend to notice but not say because of fear of the truth. I guess I can understand how my granddad felt. You go along for fear of the truth. When I think back to my granddad eating those onions, maybe that was to escape the true tears that were begging to come out without being exposed. Hmmm.

My grandma was not a good woman to me. Her treatment of me made me hate her and after what I saw she did to my grandfather, I felt like what was good for the gander was good for the goose. So, I put bleach in her insulin. This is a little boy who wanted to be free from his prison. I was done with her because she was done with me. I wanted to be free from it all and be with my mother. But man will God, look out for his children. I had done it but the insulin had turned purple, scared, I didn't go through with it. I had mixed feelings afterwards like I knew I couldn't go through with it, and I felt like I had let myself down, but I never tried anything like that again, however I did amuse myself many nights with the thoughts.

As I read this out loud from the beginning it hit differently. I realized that I still have that scared little boy locked inside, who is still hurting and afraid. This was much more difficult to write than I anticipated it would be. It makes me tear up when I reflect back. There is so much I can't go into detail about, things that I am not ready to talk about, but when I cried the first time after reading this, I realized that I am not completely healed, but I am in the healing journey. Every day I live with my past, and every day I make the decision to keep going until I reach my healing. I have been diagnosed with Cyclothymia years ago. It is a mood disorder that causes emotional highs and lows. I have often wondered if that stems from my childhood trauma which may have played a part in me sabotaging my own relationships because I didn't think I deserve to be happy. But now I accept that I do deserve to be happy and every day I do my best to stay positive and see the best in people. There are times that I am triggered, and I have to take a moment and compartmentalize the situation and deal with the here and now and not the pain of my childhood trauma. Wow, reading my story aloud brings a new perspective to my life. While it hurts to revisit the past, I know it is necessary for my healing journey.

I haven't reached a point of complete healing, but I carry the weight of my past in every interaction. I was diagnosed with cyclothymia years ago, and I often wonder if there's a connection to my childhood experiences. Do these past hurts make me sabotage my own happiness? Not anymore, I have taken back control. It feels like that more now.

Despite the challenges, I strive to stay positive and see the good in others and more importantly the good in me. Yes, I put on a brave face, hoping no one sees the turmoil within. My hope is that by sharing my story, I can encourage others to seek help, understand that it happen**ED** to you, it is not happen**ING** to you, and you have the power to be happy and you deserve to be treated with respect and you cannot make anyone treat you the way you want to be treated. If you are in any kind of relationship, rather personal, family, business and it is not healthy, you have the right to leave a be with that person or connect with that business that will treat you the way you want to be treated. Last thing, therapy is not for the weak, it is for the person who just needs to release and be released. It is a valuable resource, and it's okay to ask for it. You deserve more than a mediocre life. You are special, valued, and there are people who care about you. Remember that always! I was apprehensive about writing this chapter, but I must say that this has been very therapeutic. I have shared things I've never told anyone, in hopes that it will help someone. The tears of a black man are real. But when you wipe your tears remember this: Think what Is the best that could happen?

The Tears of a Black

Troyeusta TC Apkins

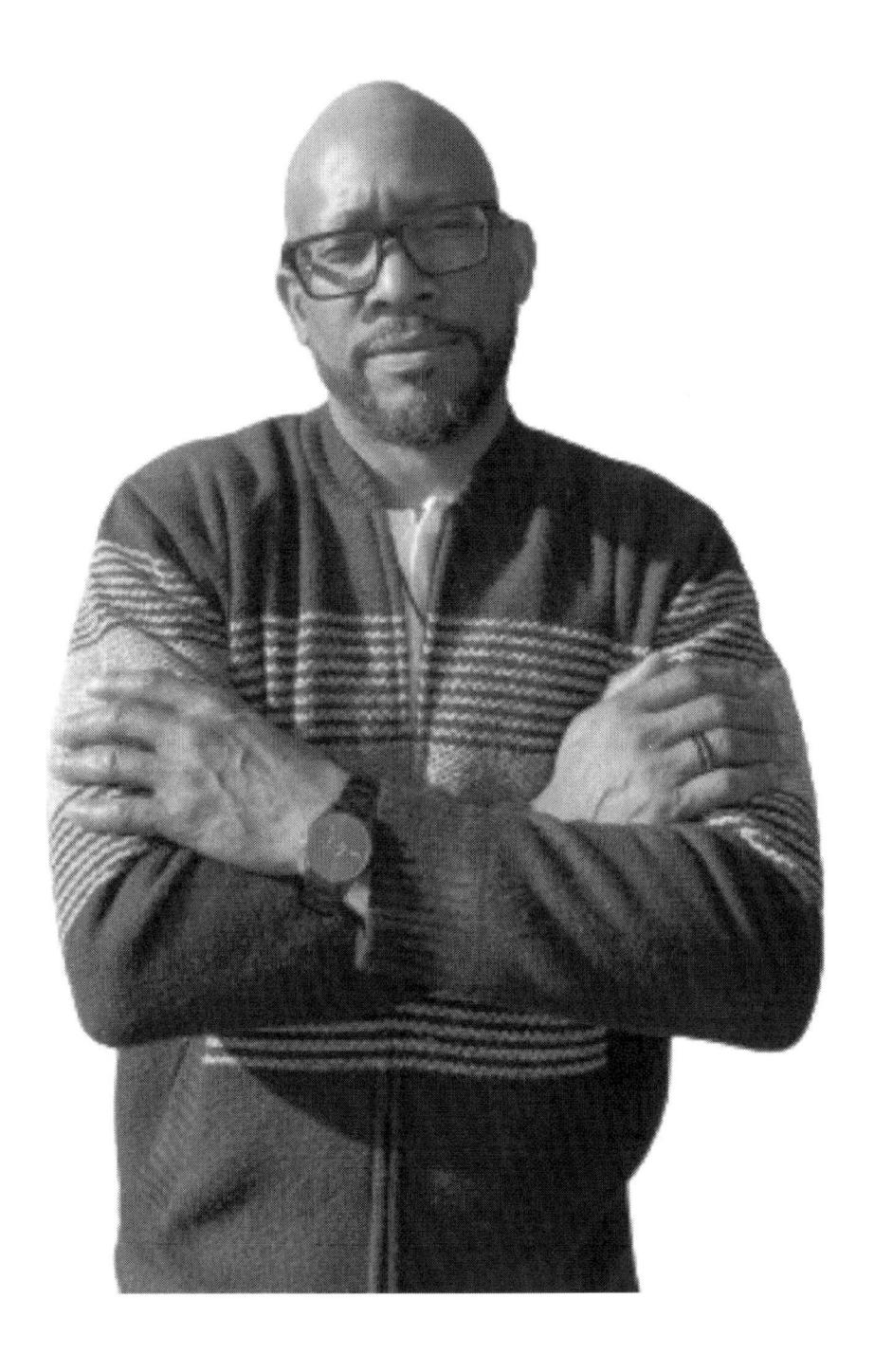

Troyeusta TC Apkins to his friends, he is known as Troy or TC, is an Alabama native. He currently resides in Georgia. He is an American actor, model, host, mentor, and now author. TC served his country in the Army as a soldier of the 82nd Airborne Division for 3 years. He is a family man, having 3 children. TC is a Law of Attraction Enthusiast and believes in positive vibes. His love for positive people, being a lover of new experiences, his gentleman charisma, and his smooth appearance on the runway has led him to be voted ATL's Hottest Male Model in 2018 and 2020.

TC's motto is: Think What's The Best That Could Happen.

WHO MADE YOU CRY

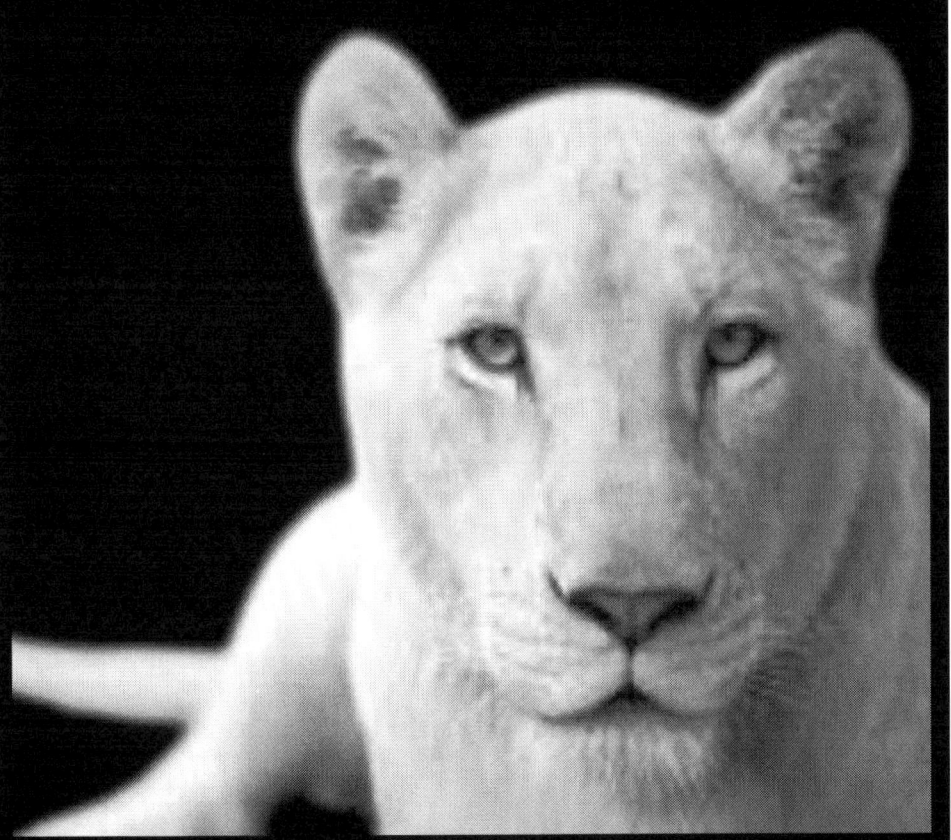

AUTHOR: SISTA JAY AJY

CHAPTER FIVE

Wait, what is a woman doing in this all-male book you may be asking? Good question, it is said that behind every good and successful man is a good woman. Well, this book is no different. I am not going to try to pretend that I understand black men or their trauma because, I am not a black man so therefore, there is no way I can understand what a black man feels the same way there is no way he can understand what I as a black woman feels however, we both can have empathy for each other.

Let me first start by saying that I am a mother of two males, I am also the daughter of a man, and the granddaughter of a man, and I am the cousin of men. I have been the wife of a man and I've had boyfriends. I have seen all of those men experience various levels of hurt, pain, mistreatment, social injustice, love loss, betrayal, deception, to state the least, so I think that I can speak from a perspective of seeing what men have gone through and have empathy for what they have experienced being a black man.

I had my first son rather young. His father hit me one time and I was out. Me leaving meant that I was now a single mother with two children. Being a mother, it was hard raising my son by myself, and I've made a lot of mistakes being a first-time male mother. I did what I thought was best based on the mindset that I had and the things that I saw. As parent's we never want to admit when we made mistakes, maybe it's because for some reason that means, we are less powerful or we are above reproach, or we just too darn stubborn to say we dropped the ball. Well, for me, I am not too proud to say, "I dropped the ball and because I dropped the ball, it had a direct impact on my son's life and how he viewed life, at least some of it was due to my ball dropping." I'm not beating up on myself, however, I am acknowledging my short comings.

What I'm about to share is very painful for me as a single mother however, it's even more painful for my oldest son to have experience it. For some you may say, "We all went through it, and you were being a parent, mines did worst." So, as I stated, I was a single mother, and although, I never saw my stepfather be physically abusive, however there was one time three of us got a whipping with a belt but somehow after my father spoke with us as to why we were getting discipline, we kinda sorta agreed we should get the whipping (well, I wasn't totally convinced but I saw his point). Nevertheless, for the most part, my stepfather was a man of words, my mother on the other hand believed in physical discipline, til this day, I shake when I see a certain type of tree. After my parents divorced and we moved to Baltimore, it had become come to see physical discipline, receive physical discipline and to see extreme discipline or harsh discipline hidden especially on boys. Even in horse playing, physical and aggressive contact was used in the name of *"I'm making you tough"*. Where I'm from boys were not allowed to cry, if they did, they would get punched. When my parents were together, if one of my brothers would cry, my father would ask them why they were crying, and just like clockwork, my father would talk with my brothers, but this was not so in Baltimore with my family and newfound friends. If a male cried because he fell or something other than death happened, he would either get punched ore joked on and women would tell him to either stop acting like a baby or crying like a girl (which was a little offensive because I was a girl and I seldom cried). So, as time progressed, I began to adapt to my environment and for a long time if I saw a man cry for any other reason than his mother or best friend or sibling dying, I viewed him as weak. Why? Because men don't cry and that meant little boys too. So, here is what I am shamefully going to share. When my son would cry because maybe he fell off of his bike and would *rightfully embrace his pain by crying*, I would order him to stop crying and if he did not, I would punch him in the chest until he stop crying, telling him to be tough. I never allowed my son to cry and if did, I popped him. My son was called a crybaby because he would cry but instead of me sitting him down and talking with him and asking him why he was crying, I used physical force to cease his crying. Even those times when I would ask him and couldn't tell me, maybe that was the time I should have comforted him as him mother and assured him everything was going to be alright. But instead, I use militant discipline to make him, force him to hide his emotions. I took away the opportunity to talk to my son on how to talk through his emotions and how to compatibilized them. Instead, I thought him how to play mascaraed and how to lie and how to not be honest with himself and how to use violence and force to solve a problem. I would buy him things to make him happy. Maybe this is why he believe money and things is the key to love and happiness and even more important why he may believe if he gives, they will love him. *(As I write this my heart hurts for my son.)* Son, in front of the world, I humbly apologize for not allowing you to embrace your emotions as a little boy. Oh, how wrong was I to take that from you. I can only pray that you will forgive me. Some may say, how could I be so open to share this with the world, well, I truly believe if we are to heal others than it first starts with home. Parents makes mistakes, some is in the name of love, and some is with malice, either way, if we are truly to be healed someone must take the first step to receive the medicine. I love my son with all my heart however, I was raising a boy child in a world that was and is dangerous. Being tough is survival and there is no room for the weak. That was my mindset. I had turned to the streets, and I surrounded myself with tough, street mentality men and women and although, now I realize and understand that my choice of parenting was improper, it was nothing compared to what I witnessed. We were young, misguided, street parents that was doing what we thought was right to keep our children from becoming prey and stay alive.

Although, I was single, I did date but to have a man live with me and my children was not a common habit. So not having a father in the house or a positive male present to influence, talk with, understand, sympathize, encourage, educate, discipline, or to just have male bonding with was very hard for my oldest son. Living in Baltimore, it was men dying every day, so for me being a mother, I was afraid for my son and the things that the world was awaiting to do to him in a society that clearly disrespects black men. It was very scary. So, I like a lot of parents did our best to raise our boys to be tough. The difference is that had I used my father's technique; the results would probably been the same without the trauma.

But I was raised in a family to where men were not allowed to cry. Men were supposed to be tough, and men were not allowed to talk about their feelings. Understand that this was never actually said out loud or directly however, we just knew it and it was implicated when the boys in my family would cry or try to express their feeling, and they were teased. So, I learned early on that men were not supposed to feel. I learned early on that men were not supposed to cry. I learned early on that men were supposed to be tough, and I learned early on that little boys were supposed to be little men, and I indirectly passed that on to my children.

I later learned in life that that wasn't fair. How could you expect for a little boy to be a man when he has yet to experience being a little boy? How can you expect for a little boy to have the courage of a full grown man when he is yet to overcome the fear of walking to bathroom in the dark? How can you expect the little boy to hold back his tears when he has been hurt? That's not fair, and it wasn't fair to my oldest son.

Society has taught us that men do not have permission to embrace their trauma. So they go through life, living a lie.

Little boys are not made of snakes, and snails and puppy dog tails. (I believe that nursey rhyme was made up by some woman that was mistreat or abused by her husband and she made is up while singing to her child and it just caught on. But I digress). Boys are human and they feel just like little girls. They are not machine made with a bunch of instructions; they are trying to figure it out just like the girls. So why is it that we put the pressure of manhood on a boy? We expect them to be something they have no clue to what it means to be. Boys have hormones confusion just like girls. The have emotionally, and mental break downs and *unsurieties* just like their counterparts. So, why in the world would we expect for a little boy think like or act like a grown man? It's not fair.

We teach our little boys at a very young age to compartmentalize their emotions and not to show them but just like a tea kettle it will eventually blow and if that little boy has not been given proper guidance on how to deal with his emotions, in most cases it does not turn out well. So, we setup them up for failure after failure because when little boys grow up and get into relationships, women are expecting for them to show emotions and relate to them on some levels. But how can they when they have been desensitized to their emotions? Our little boys become grown men that have been brainwashed to hide their emotions and if they share their emotions, they believed that they are looked at as a wimp, or a punk, or being soft. Yes, men are not going to walking around just laying their feelings out, but men should have a safe place to vent their emotions and or trauma out and not be judged for it.

Is it true that all little boys are supposed to play some type of sports like football, basketball, or baseball? But what about the little boy who does not have an interest in sports? Does that make weak or less of a boy or man? Society says if a man does not do certain things as a male, then that male is not a real boy. So if he's not a boy what is he? We have to stop this buffoonery of what society says a little boy should be or how a male should at. Every male does not want to be the biggest, and baddest muncho man. Some males just want to be chilled. There should be a balance for men just like there is a balance for women. Every man is not tough, just like every woman is not soft. Just because you see that a man is not from the rough parts of the track doesn't mean he is any less of a man. Just because he doesn't want to shoot somebody or pick a fight doesn't mean he doesn't have heart. I'm not sure where the concept of he is not big, bad and tough, he is a whimp comes from, but I can tell you that there are a lot of big, bad, tough men in the graves and in prison for life.

Little boys like my son who were not allowed to embrace that instead little boy, grow up with rage inside of them because they were not taught how to release it and they make detrimental mistakes on top of detrimental mistakes, hurting themselves, and others seeking for a way to deal with their emotions and or trauma.

In the last few years, women have been speaking out in the 'Me Too' movement against some high-profile celebrities. In that movement, there are a few men that have spoken out. What is sadly amazing to me is that rather on a high-profile level or in elementary schools, males are being assaulted just as much as females are, but it is not reported due to the stigma attached to it or the shame of a male not being able to defend himself. So, now we have not unhealed traumatized women but unhealed traumatized men trying to live. I can't say one assault is worse than the other because both is a violation of a person. The only difference is that women have been given permission to embrace their pain (if they so choose to) more easily than a man. Society says that rape of a woman is acceptable violation, but rape of a male should not be spoken of and if it is, then the male is somehow viewed a gay or weak. (How so unfair) So, these males go through life not having a safe place to release their hurt, pain and violation without the predator's condemnation being placed on the victim. Violated men have not been given permission to embrace what happened to them and to say, this happened to me without the shameful stares. In a time when he would need to support of his most trust friends and loved ones, the fear of them judging him, turning their backs on him leaves him living in unhealed trauma, causing his character to be of negativity.

I have had the fortitude of talking with men that have been violated. When I stated that I would be writing this book, there were some things they wanted me to share in hopes of their fellow brothers having non-judgmental empathy. To protect names and their privacy I will not use names as I share their story.

There was a middle school male student that was always told he was handsome. His teachers all loved him. One day he stayed after school to help one of his female teachers. She left out the classroom for a few moments and returned back to the classroom. He noticed she had locked the door, and she went to the part of the classroom that could not be seen through the glass of the door. She asked him to come help her. He said he couldn't remember what it was, but he went over to her. He said he remembered her touching his butt and giggling. She told him his butt was soft. She asked him if he thought she was pretty. He said he nervously shook his head yes. She asked him if he wanted to suck her breast. He was shocked. He said he didn't know what to do. So, he froze. She pulled him near him, and bend down unbutton, and unzipped his pants, and began to perform fellatio on him. Of course, he said he like it, but he was scared and confused. His teacher was giving him head, a grown woman was having oral sex with a thirteen-year-old boy. When she finished, she pulled up her dress, turned around, bend over, and helped him enter inside of her. Once she finished, she yelled for him to get out and he better not tell a soul, or she would scream rape. When he came back to school the next day, she acted as if nothing happened, in fact he said she was rather short with him. He said remember thinking maybe she didn't like him, or he did it wrong. But to his surprise, she asked him to stay back after school and it was a repeat. He said this continued for the remainder of the school year. He said that it messed with his mind because of how she would treat him and the more they did it he would do his best to please her so she wouldn't be made at him the next day. So, in his mind, he felt as if all women were like that. He said that when he did finally tell his boys that summer, they didn't see what the problem was, and they wished it happened to him. The next school year, he said she wouldn't even look at him. He shared with me, that he doesn't talk about it because society doesn't deem what he went through as a trauma but for him it was. He states that it is hard for him to genuinely love a woman. Although, it wasn't vicious, it was still a trauma that he has yet to deal with. He did state that by talking with me and me not judging him, and really having empathy for him helped him.

The next fella story, shared with me his abandonment issues. He stated that one day he came home for high school and his mother had packed up and left. Just like that, she had left him. When I asked him what he did, he stated that he told his grandmother. His grandmother said that his mother went to live with her boyfriend and that he could come stay with her or stay there since it was government housing until the lease had to be signed. At first, he said he was hurt, but then he liked the idea of being at home with no one telling him what to do. He then said from nowhere he stated feeling a since of loneliness and emptiness. He said that when the lease was up, he went to stay with his grandmother, and from that point he would always live with a woman until they broke up or they put him out. He said he found himself dealing with a lot of demeaning stuff, just to stay with the woman. He said that he always kept a job, and he had descent credit so getting a place of his own wasn't the issue. After a long conversation, he admitted because his father had left him and his mother, and then his mother left him, he had abandonment issues. So, he put up with a lot of bull and chose women that was needed so he wouldn't be abandoned. He soon got his own house and now he is working through his issues in therapy. Again, I shared these stories so that you can see that everyone has something that they are dealing with that makes them not okay, and that's okay but what is not okay is doing something about it. Men have life happening just like women, maybe on a different scale but it's still happening and it's okay to embrace it in order to overcome it.

Although, society says men don't suppose to cry, there are a few times when a man is allowed to cry. As crazy as it may sound, sports are a man's pass to cry or feel emotions. Why is it that men are more comfortable showing emotions for a game that consist of a bunch of strangers than they do with their loved ones? Again, this is a language that only a man can answer (and is this is not just a black thing). I wonder if this is so because men feel safe in sports. Could this be their safe place where they can show their emotions both negative and positive and not be judged for it? Hmmm, as a woman, I wonder.

Mental illness is a real thing. I believe now that so many white people loved ones have committed suicide, it is okay to talk about. But black men have been dealing with mental illness for a long time, some of is contributed to chemical imbalance and some is due to the tumor of society. Because black men, are viewed as weak if they say they need help, they shut down and turn to the bottle, drugs, sex, or violence to suppress their issues. The mind is a powerful organ, and it can hold a lot however, after a while if the mind is not given the opportunity to release some of the weight it is carrying, it will shut down or go haywire. You owe it to yourself to decompress and release. You owe it to yourself to get to your safe place and let it out and sometimes a good cry is all you need.

I'm hoping that after reading this book it will begin some type of dialogue amongst black men to create that safe space so that they can express their feelings in hopes of healing, and to be a better them. It is so true that hurting people hurt people, but loving people love people too.

I will continue to pray that your ailing hearts will turn into healing hearts so that it can embrace love at its fullest, because the story behind the tears of a black man is strong, powerful, prosperous, overcoming, victorious, loving, yes Godly.

SISTA JAY JAY

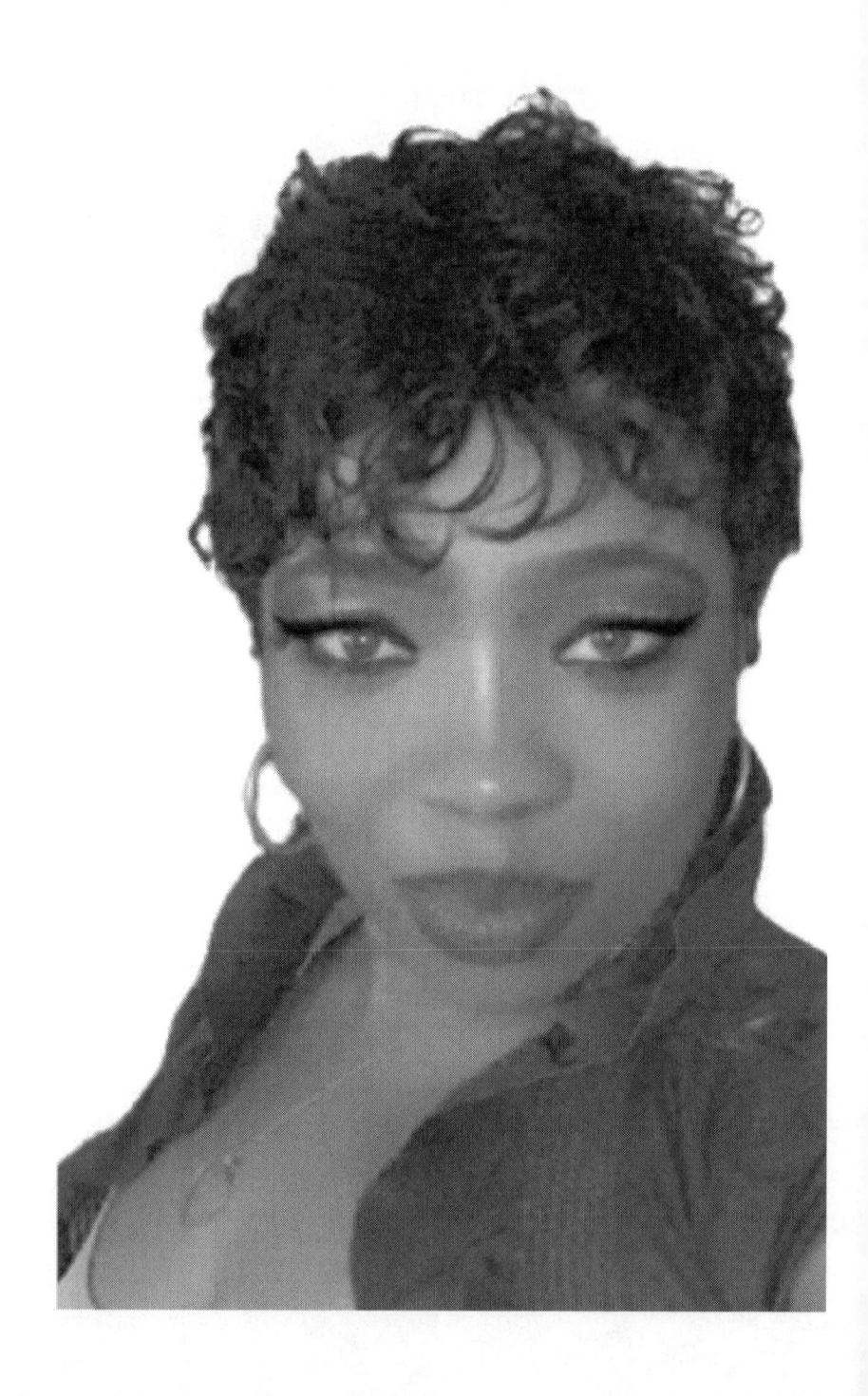

Sista Jay Jay (JoeDrell Benjamin) native of Petersburg, Virginia by way of Baltimore Maryland, currently resides in Georgia. Sista Jay Jay is an executive producer, director, screenwriter, playwright, actor, artist, a self-published author, podcastor, philanthropist, and a businesswoman. She has worked as an actor, writer, director and producer for over 20 years in the entertainment industry. She has written, directed and produced over a dozen stage play productions, (listed on her IMDb). Added to her credit is one short film "Crazy on Another Level", three independent films, "Too Crazy on Another Level", (IMDb credited) now streaming on Tubi, Amazon Prime and Stash TV, 'Men Pray Too" (IMDb credited), now streaming on Tubi and Hoopla, Plex, LG, Viz. One web series, "Side Chick Chronicles"(IMDb credited), one docu-series "#Black Men Vote", What Would You Do (streaming 2024).

Sista Jay Jay is also credited on Amazon for nine books under her Publishing company, R.A.G Girl

Publishing, she has two R.A.G Girl Best selling collaborations books, A Love Story vol. 1 Why I call him lover, vol. 2 My Journey to Love. She is a best-selling collaboration author for a collaboration book Love, Life and Lock Up, Vol. 4 with Michelle Lovett. Her single, The Queen is here-The Boss Lady Anthem is currently streaming on all music platforms.

Sista Jay Jay was the editor and chief of two publications, B.O.S.S Magazine and King Up Magazine and is the CEO of Qween Body Care. She owns, A Sip of Jay drink company. Sista is the creator and host of her podcast, 'Everybody got something to say' (YouTube; Sista Jay Jay Tv), The Diamond Girlz Talk, and she is also co-host on DC Curry's podcast, DisRace (YouTube; DC Curry Tv). Sista Jay Jay is an acting coach (A.B.C-Actors Boot Camp Workshop). Her award-winning production company, No Nykel n Dyme Production has contributed to bringing several filmmaker's visions to film. When she is not working, Sista Jay Jay hosts two yearly charity events, Models Against Cancer and Models Against Hunger along with several other charitable events under her non-profit organization, The Bridging hand Inc. Sista Jay Jay is a mentor, motivational speaker, and certified life coach. She hosts two annual conferences, Sista Jay Jay's Brunch with the Queens in Georgia and Real Men will Talk and Gentlemen's recognition in Georgia.

She is an honorary member with the Elite Dollz of Faith LLC for her selfless contribution to helping others and 2023 Women of Honor recipient.

She will be releasing her third volume from the collaboration book series, A Love Story vol. 3 The Price I Paid in September 2024.

Sista Jay Jay lives by the motto, "Be the best that you can be because no one is better at being you than you". Her work ethic motto is WWW; willingness + Work=Winners.

She loves God and God's people.

For Sista Jay Jay, it is not about being right as much as it is about getting it right.

You can find Sista Jay Jay on all social media at: I Am Sista Jay Jay.

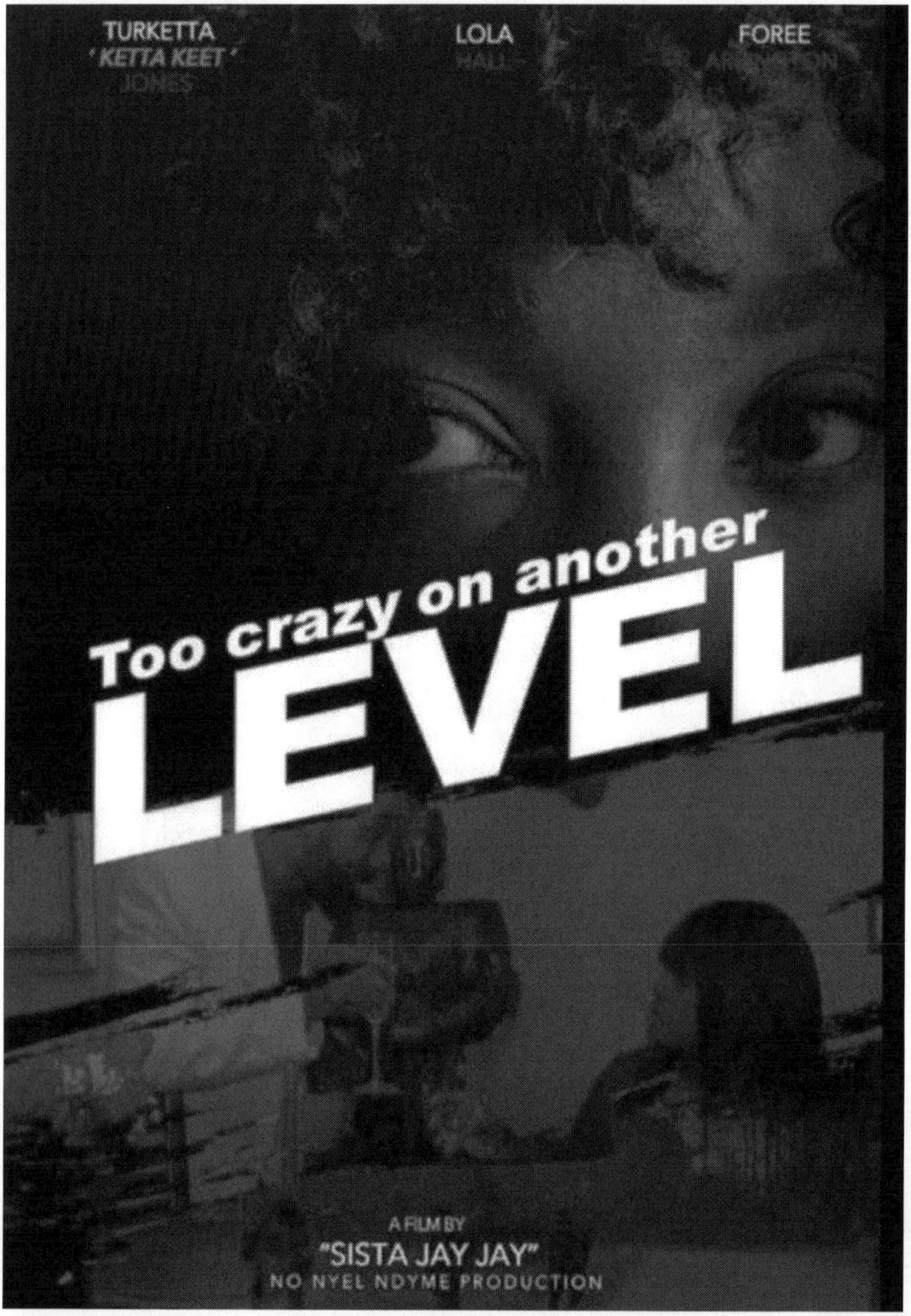
TURKETTA
' KETTA KEET '
JONES
LOLA
HALL
FOREE
Too crazy on another
LEVEL
A FILM BY
"SISTA JAY JAY"
NO NYEL NDYME PRODUCTION

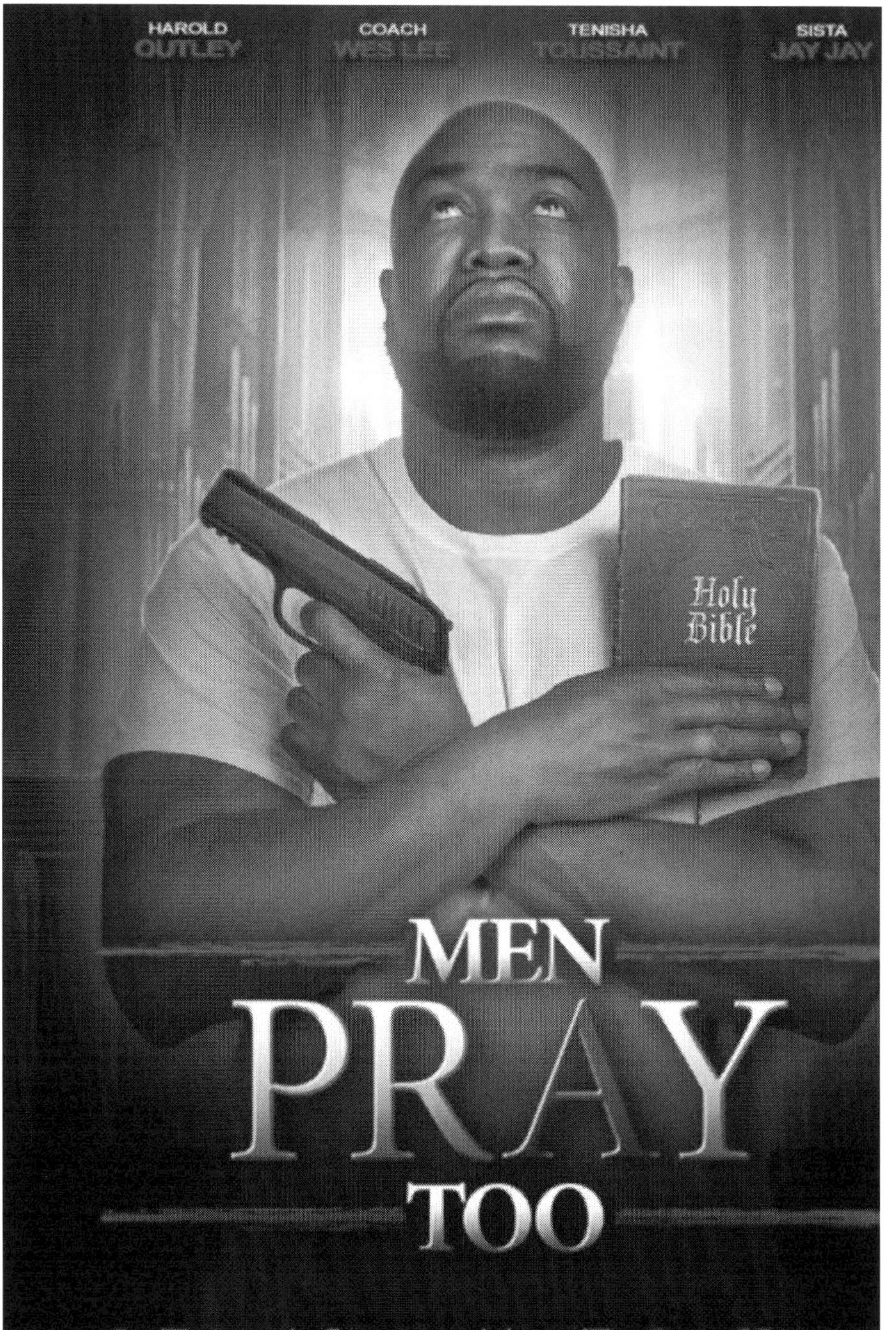
HAROLD
OUTLEY
COACH
WES LEE
TENISHA
TOUSSAINT
SISTA
JAY JAY
Holy
Bible
MEN
PRAY
TOO
IT TAKES A STRONG MAN TO SAVE HIMSELF

The Tears of a Black

Made in the USA
Columbia, SC
11 June 2024